SPORTS SUPPLEMENTS

WHAT NUTRITIONAL
SUPPLEMENTS REALLY WORK

D0774805

, 2007   0713682590

SPORTS SUPPLEMENTS

WHAT NUTRITIONAL SUPPLEMENTS REALLY WORK

Anita Bean

A & C Black • London

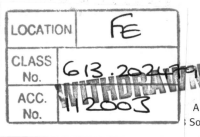
First published 2007 by
A & C Black Publishers Ltd
Soho Square, London W1D 3HB
www.acblack.com

ISBN-13: 978 0 7136 8259 5

The right of Anita Bean to be identified as the author of this work has been asserted by her in accordance with the Copyright, Designs and Patents Act 1988

A CIP catalogue record for this book is available from the British Library.

Note: The information contained in this book is presented for educational purposes only and should not be construed as medical advice. The content of this book is not meant in any way to substitute, contradict, or replace specific health recommendations from your doctor or health professional, nor should it be used to diagnose, treat, cure or prevent any disease.

Cover design by Jocelyn Lucas
Text design by Mark Roberts at Talking Design
Cover photographs courtesy of © istockphoto.com
Inside photographs courtesy of istockphoto.com and shutterstock.com

This book is produced using paper that is made from wood grown in managed, sustainable forests. It is natural, renewable and recyclable. The logging and manufacturing processes conform to the environmental regulations of the country of origin.

Typeset in MetaPlusNormal by Palimpsest Book Production Limited, Grangemouth, Stirlingshire
Printed and bound in Spain by GraphyCems

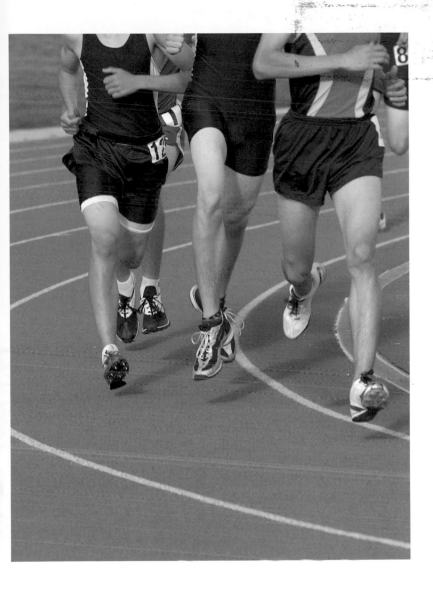

CONTENTS

INTRODUCTION

I wrote this guide in response to the growing public confusion, hype and controversy surrounding sports supplements. With more than 2000 products and at least 40 different brands to choose from in the United Kingdom, separating hype and fact isn't easy. We spend £180 million a year on sports nutrition products, according to a 2006 Datamonitor report, including £41 million on sports supplements. My aim is to try to clarify the information about sports supplements and provide you with relevant and balanced advice to help you make informed decisions. The result is an independent evaluation of the most popular sports supplements.

– Anita Bean

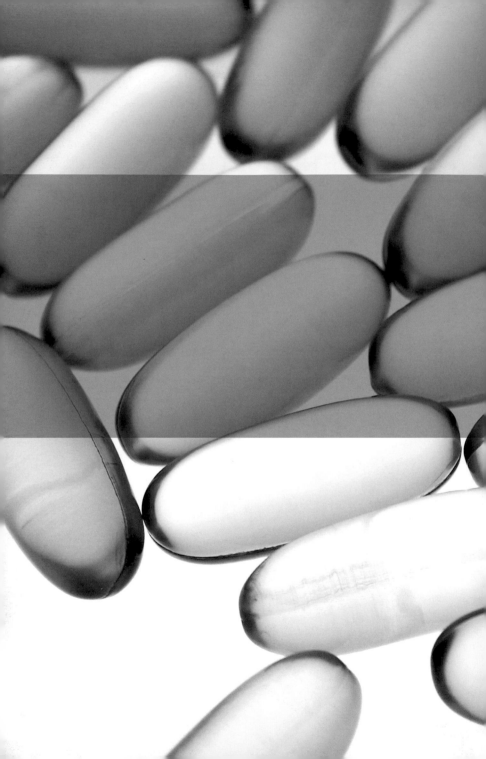

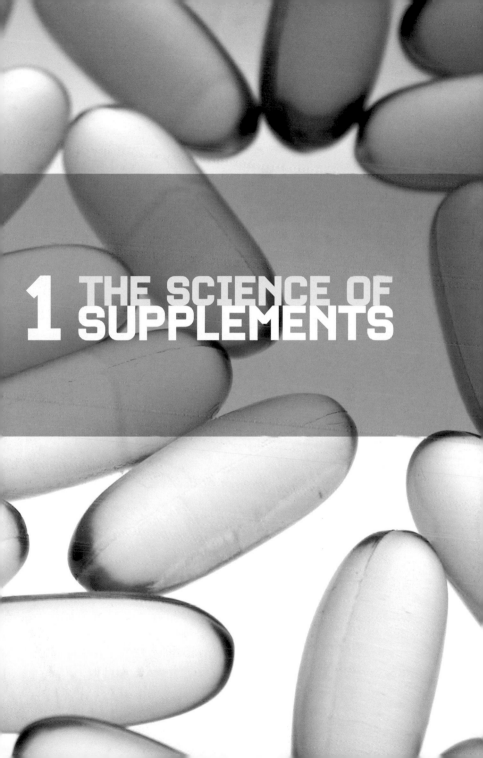

1 THE SCIENCE OF SUPPLEMENTS

WHAT ARE SPORTS SUPPLEMENTS?

Sports supplements are a category of nutritional supplements, concentrated sources of nutrients or other substances with a nutritional or physiological effect whose purpose is to supplement the normal diet. They are marketed to athletes, sports people and active people for improving physical performance, and include tablets, capsules, powders, drinks and bars.

Many athletes believe supplements are an essential component for sports success and it has been estimated that the majority of elite athletes are using some form of performance-enhancing agent. A US study of collegiate varsity athletes found that 65 per cent used supplements regularly, while a similar Canadian study revealed that 99 per cent of varsity athletes used supplements either regularly or intermittently. The most popular varieties are multivitamins, followed by carbohydrate/energy supplements, protein supplements, creatine and caffeine. Ephedrine, androstenedione, glutamine and HMB are also popular among strength athletes.

But the use of supplements is not essential for progress. Your dietary needs can be met through the preparation of a well-tailored diet (*see* 'Sports nutrition', page 21).

WHAT'S SAFE?

There is currently no specific European or national legislation governing the safety of sports supplements. Sports supplements are classified as foods, so they are not subject to the same strict manufacturing, safety testing or labelling requirements as licensed medicines. This means that there is no guarantee that a supplement lives up to its claims. At the time of going to print, the European Union (EU) is reviewing the situation with a view to introducing stricter labelling requirements in the future.

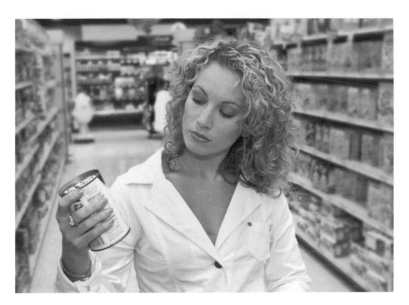

However, there is stricter legislation covering vitamin and mineral supplements (the EU Food Supplements Directive, 2002, amended August 2005). Manufacturers can only use nutrients and ingredients from a 'permitted' list, and then within maximum limits. Each ingredient must undergo extensive safety tests before it is allowed on the permitted list and, therefore, into a supplement. Manufacturers must also provide scientific proof to support a product's claims and ensure that it is clearly labelled.

WHAT'S LEGAL?

Tests have found that some sports supplements do not always contain the ingredients declared on the label; others may be contaminated with prohibited stimulants or substances.

A 2001 survey, by the International Olympic Committee-accredited laboratory in Cologne, of 634 supplements found 15 per cent contained banned substances, including nandrolone (*see* 'Pre-hormones/ prohormones', page 105). Nineteen per cent of UK samples were contaminated. Another study in 2000 at the Olympic Analytical

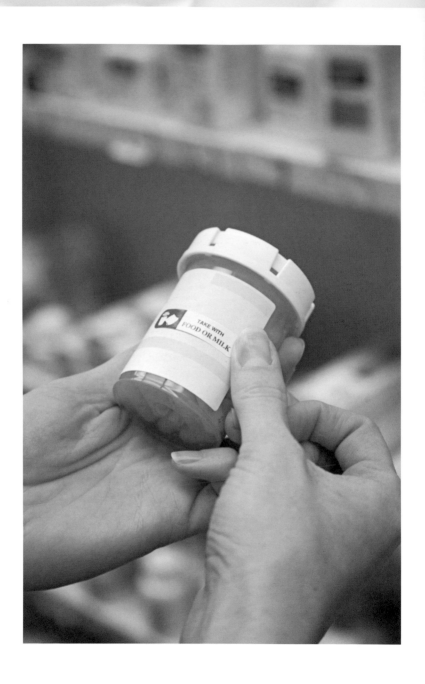

Laboratory at the University of California found some brands of androstenedione were grossly mis-labelled and contained the illegal anabolic steroid, testosterone. In 2001, Swiss researchers found different substances from those declared on the labels, including testosterone, in 7 out of 17 pro-hormone supplements, i.e. 41 per cent of the sample.

ADVICE TO UK ATHLETES ON THE USE OF SUPPLEMENTS

In light of concerns about contamination and poor labelling of supplements, UK Sport, the British Olympic Association, the British Paralympic Association, the National Sports Medicine Institute and the home country Sports Councils advise UK athletes to be 'extremely cautious' about the use of any supplement, including vitamins, minerals, ergogenic aids and herbal remedies. They warn about the possible risk of contamination and advise that supplements are taken at the athlete's own risk (anti-doping rules are based on the principle of strict liability).

Athlete's must sign a code of conduct agreeing that they are responsible for what they take, but they are advised to consult a medical practitioner, accredited sports dietitian or registered nutritionist before taking any supplements

WHAT'S LEGAL

The following substances are banned by the International Olympic Committee (IOC) and would result in a positive drugs test:

- 19-Norandrostenediol
- 19-Norandrostenedione
- Androstenediol
- Androstenedione
- Dehydroepiandrosterone (DHEA)
- Ephedrine
- Strychnine

HOW TO EVALUATE A SUPPLEMENT

- Don't be taken in by supplements that promise dramatic results. If the manufacturer's claims sound too good to be true, then they probably are.
- Be sceptical of advertisements that contain lots of technical jargon, unnecessary graphs or big words. If the information isn't clear and factual, leave the supplement well alone.

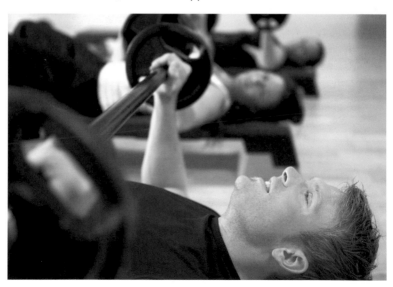

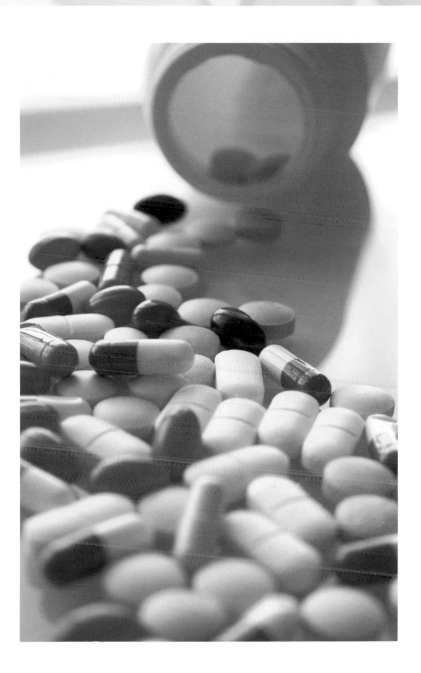

- Be wary of glossy advertisements that rely on astonishing 'before and after' photos rather than scientifically sound evidence for the supplement.
- Ask the manufacturer for evidence and/or studies that support the supplement's claims. If the information isn't available, don't touch the supplement.
- Check that any evidence is unbiased. Ideally, studies should have been carried out at a university, published in a reputable scientific journal and should not have been funded solely by the manufacturer.
- Don't take a supplement that has been recommended only by word of mouth. Check out exactly what's in it and whether it works before you buy it. Ask an expert if you have any questions.

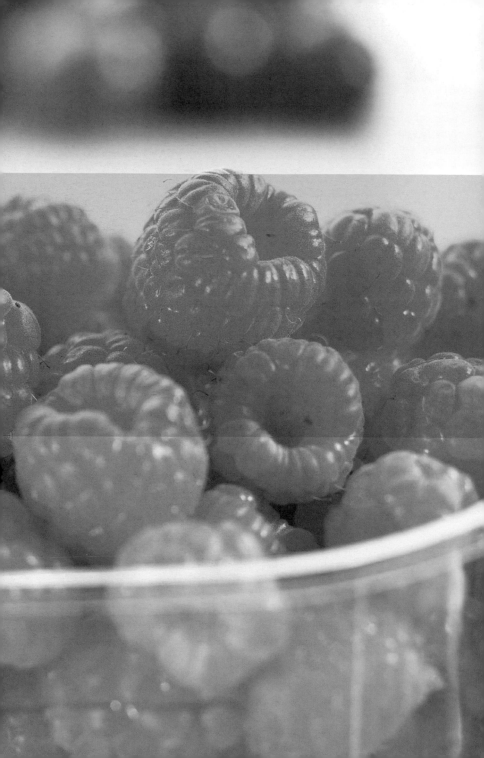

2 SPORTS SUPPLEMENT CATEGORIES

Sports supplements can be categorised according to their main mode of action (although there is some overlap between categories):

- muscle mass and strength
- energy and endurance
- recovery after exercise.

MUSCLE MASS AND STRENGTH

"ALL-IN-ONE" OR "COMBINATION SUPPLEMENTS"

These usually take Protein Powders or MRPs as a base and add specialist supplements such as creatine, glutamine or HMB into a single supplement.

AMINO ACIDS

Amino acids are the building blocks of protein. These supplements, including branched chain amino acids, are popular with athletes during intense training periods who sometimes prefer this method to protein shakes.

CREATINE

Creatine may help increase your strength and muscle mass by allowing you to train at maximum intensity for a little longer. Creatine has been studied extensively by scientists and is widely used by sprint, power and strength athletes to improve performance.

MEAL REPLACEMENT PRODUCTS (MRPs)

These contain a mixture of carbohydrates, protein (usually whey and casein), vitamins and minerals and other nutrients. MRPs provide a well-balanced and convenient alternative to solid food. They are tailored towards aiding muscular growth and recovery.

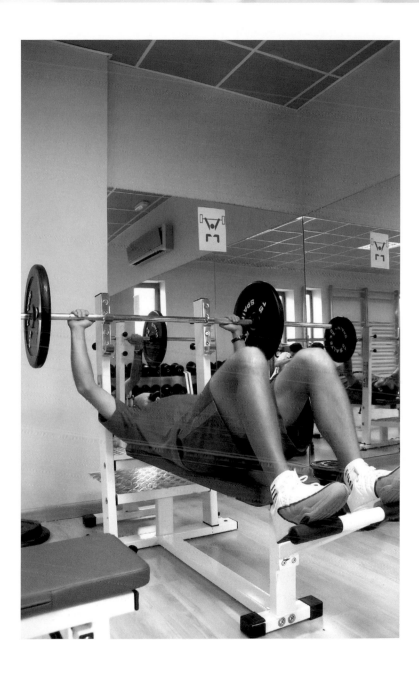

PROTEIN SUPPLEMENTS

Intense exercise increases your need for protein, so protein supplements may help meet your daily requirement and, therefore, help strength athletes to maintain or gain muscle mass. They come in three forms: protein powders, ready-to-drink formulas and high-protein nutrition bars.

OTHER SUPPLEMENTS IN THIS CATEGORY INCLUDE:

- Androstenedione
- Glutamine
- HMB
- Pre-hormones
- ZMA.

ENERGY AND ENDURANCE

SPORTS DRINKS

Isotonic sports drinks aim to replace fluid during and after exercise, as well as provide carbohydrate fuel for exercising muscles. They also contain electrolytes (sodium and potassium) to help your body better retain the fluid.

ENERGY BARS

Energy bars provide a convenient energy source before, during and after intense exercise.

ENERGY DRINKS

Energy drinks provide higher levels of carbohydrate than regular sports drinks. Generally, between 12 and 20 g per 100 ml is particularly useful for very intense workouts lasting more than 60 minutes. Energy drinks help maintain blood sugar levels, fuel muscles, and slow down the rate of glycogen depletion.

ENERGY GELS

Energy gels provide a highly concentrated source of carbohydrates. Consumed during endurance exercise lasting more than 60 minutes, they can help delay fatigue and improve endurance.

CAFFEINE

This central nervous system stimulant can increase concentration, alertness and endurance. It raises blood levels of fatty acids, which can fuel exercising muscles and spare muscle glycogen.

OTHER SUPPLEMENTS IN THIS CATEGORY INCLUDE:

- Ephedrine/Ma huang
- Fat burners or thermogenics
- Ginseng.

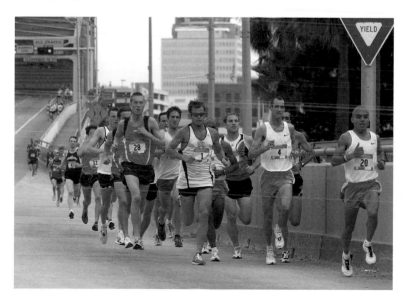

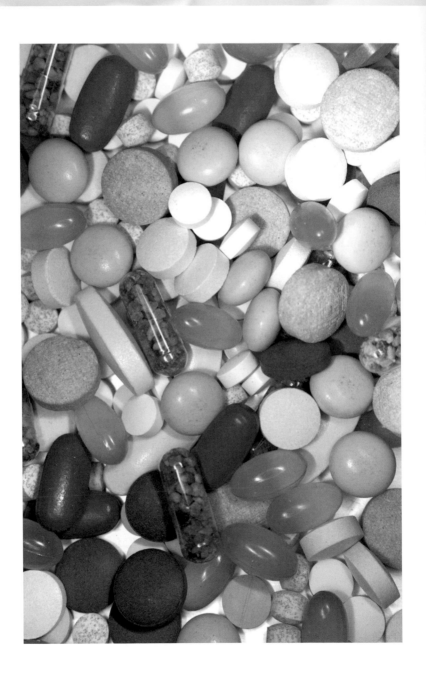

RECOVERY

NUTRITION BARS

Nutrition bars provide a convenient source of carbohydrate, protein, vitamins and minerals. They can help refuel the muscles and aid recovery.

MULTIVITAMIN AND MINERAL SUPPLEMENTS

These can help promote 'optimal' levels of vitamins and minerals to support health and performance. Most regular exercisers would probably benefit from taking a supplement.

ANTIOXIDANT SUPPLEMENTS

These may give you increased protection from heart disease and cancer, as well as promoting recovery after intense exercise and reducing post-exercise muscle soreness.

FISH OILS AND OTHER OMEGA 3 RICH SUPPLEMENTS

These may help reduce inflammation, pain and joint stiffness, promote post-workout recovery, and optimise aerobic performance.

GLUCOSAMINE AND CHONDROITIN

These supplements help maintain mobility, repair damaged cartilage, and reduce joint pain and inflammation.

OTHER SUPPLEMENTS IN THIS CATEGORY INCLUDE:

- Energy drinks
- Glutamine
- Sports drinks.

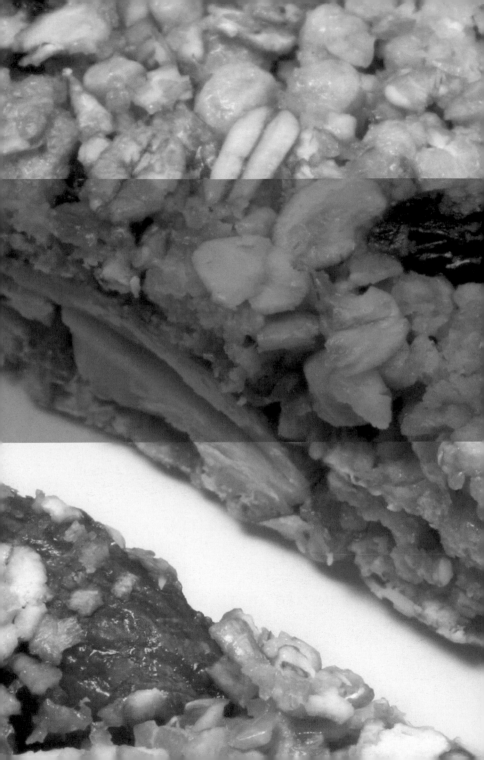

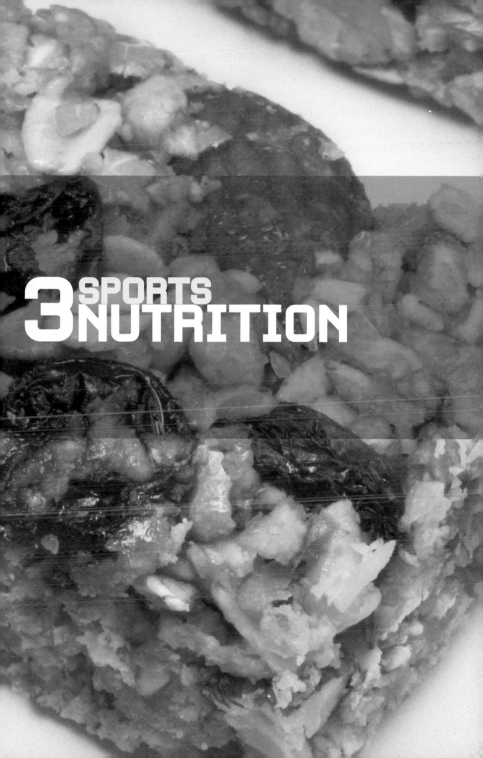

3 SPORTS NUTRITION

Good nutrition is a crucial part of every exercise programme. Whether you workout regularly to keep fit, train with weights, or take part in competitive sports, you need a healthy diet tailored to your exercise regime. What, how much and when you eat and drink makes a big difference to your performance. A healthy diet can increase your energy and endurance, reduce fatigue, maximise your strength and muscle gains, speed recovery, and improve your body composition. This section provides you with a useful practical guide to help you put together your daily training diet.

When it comes to planning your food intake, it is helpful to break the rules down into three distinct periods of time – before training, during training and after training.

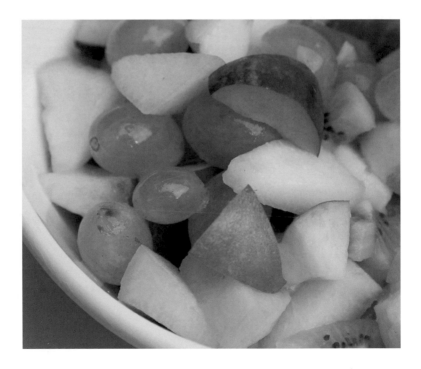

BEFORE TRAINING

WHAT TO EAT

Ideally, you should have a light meal 2–4 hours before your workout, according to a study at the University of North Carolina, USA. This will allow you to exercise longer and perform better.

Eating slow-burning or low-GI meals will produce a gradual rise in blood sugar levels, help spare muscle glycogen, and avoid problems of low blood sugar levels during long training sessions, according to studies at the University of Sydney, Australia.

Eating protein or fat with a high-GI carbohydrate will lower its GI. For example, a slice of bread with butter or cheese has a lower GI than bread on its own.

PRE-WORKOUT MEALS (TO BE EATEN 2-4 HOURS BEFORE EXERCISE)

- Sandwich/roll/bagel/wrap filled with chicken, fish, cheese, egg or peanut butter
- Jacket potato with beans, cheese, tuna, coleslaw or chicken
- Pasta with tomato-based pasta sauce and cheese
- Rice or other grains with chicken or fish and vegetables
- Porridge made with milk
- Wholegrain cereal (e.g. bran or wheat flakes, muesli or Weetabix) with milk or yoghurt.

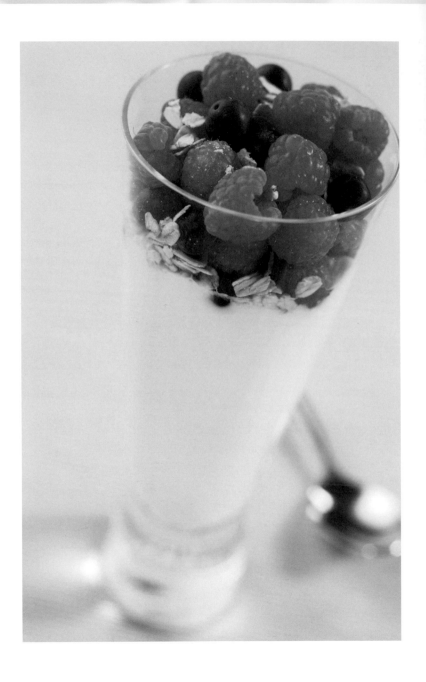

PRE-WORKOUT SNACKS (TO BE EATEN 1 - 2 HOURS BEFORE EXERCISE)

- Fresh fruit
- Dried apricots or sultanas
- Smoothie (homemade or ready-bought)
- Yoghurt
- Shake (homemade or a commercial meal replacement shake)
- Energy/cereal/breakfast bar (without hydrogenated fat)
- Fruit loaf or raisin bread

WHAT TO DRINK

Watching your urine is the best way to check your body's hydration. Dark, gold-coloured urine is a sure sign that you're low on fluid. Drink plenty of water and aim for light, yellow-coloured urine.

Drink before you get thirsty. By the time your thirst mechanism kicks in you will have lost around 2 per cent of your body weight as water.

Drink at least two glasses of water (400–600 ml) 2–3 hours before your workout. This is the amount recommended by the American College of Sports Medicine. Also ensure you carry a bottle of water with you everywhere you go.

Have a glass of water first thing in the morning and then schedule drink stops during your day. Aim for at least eight glasses ($1\frac{1}{2}$–2 l) daily, and more in hot weather or workout days.

DURING TRAINING

WHAT TO EAT

For most activities lasting less than an hour, knocking back anything other than water is unnecessary. But if you are planning to exercise for

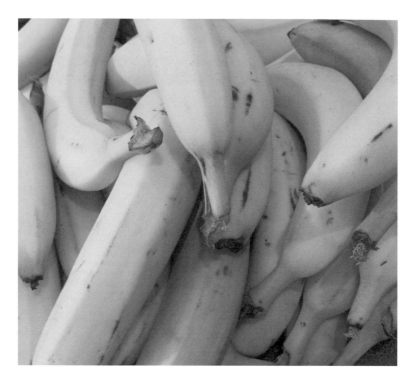

longer than 1 hour, consuming 30–60 g carbohydrate per hour can help you keep going longer. This carbohydrate helps to keep your blood sugar levels steady and fuels your muscles, particularly in the latter stages of your workout when glycogen reserves are likely to be low.

Eat little and often – your goal is to maintain a steady supply of carbohydrate entering your bloodstream. Aim to consume 15–30 g every 30 minutes.

Choose fast-burning high- or moderate-GI carbohydrates, as you need to get the carbohydrates into your bloodstream rapidly. Drinks containing sugar, glucose and maltodextrin (glucose polymers) would be suitable, but solid foods work equally well, according to one study at Cornell University, USA.

WORKOUT FOODS (WHEN TRAINING FOR LONGER THAN 60 MINUTES)

Note: Eat these with plenty of water:

- energy, cereal or breakfast bar
- energy gel
- dried fruit – raisins, sultanas, apricots or dates
- bananas
- biscuits – fig rolls, Jaffa cakes and digestives
- chocolate
- fruit cake or malt loaf.

The sizes of bars, gels and biscuits vary. Check the carbohydrate content on the label to work out how much you'll need to supply 30–60 g per hour. Choose products that supply less than 5 g fat per portion.

WHAT TO DRINK

Losing the equivalent of 2 per cent of your body weight as sweat – that's a mere 1.3 kg loss if you weigh 65 kg – results in a 10–20 per cent drop in your performance (i.e. aerobic capacity).

The American College of Sports Medicine and American Dietetics Association recommend drinking 150–350 ml every 15–20 minutes, or according to your thirst. If you can only manage a few sips at a time, then make sure you do that frequently, say every 10 minutes.

You should start drinking early during your workout as it takes about 30 minutes for the fluid to be absorbed into your bloodstream. Don't wait until you feel really thirsty as this indicates that you are already on your way to dehydration!

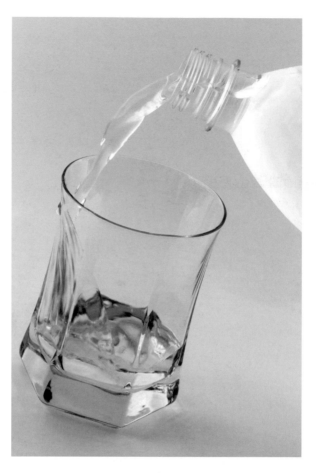

If you are aiming to lose body fat, drink plain water during your workout. Sports drinks add extra calories and, in some cases, may even supply as many, or more, calories as you are burning off!

Workouts lasting less than 1 hour

For most activities, water is all you need. It is absorbed relatively fast into your bloodstream, so does a very good job at keeping your body hydrated. It's cheap, plentiful and readily available. If you're not keen

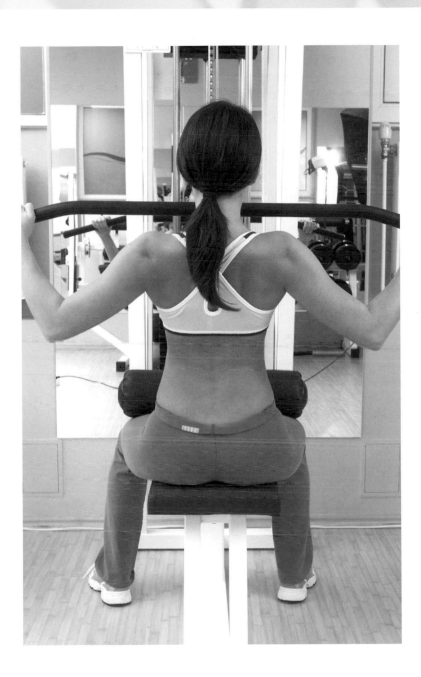

on the taste and cannot force enough down, flavour it with a little cordial, fruit juice or high-juice squash. Obviously, any kind of squash or juice contributes extra sugar (carbohydrate) but, provided it's well diluted, this won't harm your performance.

Workouts lasting more than 1 hour

Sports drinks, energy drinks, diluted juice and high-juice squash are often a better choice than plain water when you are working out continually for longer than 60 minutes. The sugars in these drinks not only provide fuel for your exercising muscles, but they also speed up the absorption of water into your bloodstream. Aim to consume 30–60 g of carbohydrate per hour – that's equivalent to 500 ml–1 l of an isotonic sports drink (containing 6 g sugar per 100 ml) or fruit juice diluted 50/50 with water.

AFTER TRAINING

WHAT TO EAT

Amazingly, it's after – not during – your workout when your body gets stronger and fitter. So what and how much you eat post-exercise is important.

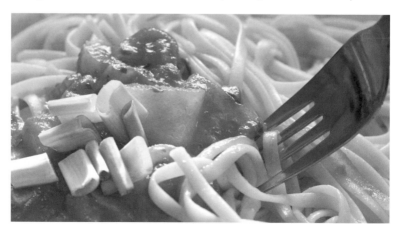

Carbohydrate helps your muscles to recover after exercise and provides the fuel needed for your next workout. It is also converted into glycogen one-and-a-half times faster than normal during the 2 hours after training.

POST-WORKOUT SNACKS

(To be eaten within 2 hours after exercise)

- A couple of pieces of fresh fruit with a glass of milk
- 1 or 2 cartons of yoghurt
- A smoothie (crushed fresh fruit whizzed in a blender)
- A homemade milkshake
- A yoghurt drink
- Flavoured milk
- A sports bar
- A tuna or cottage cheese sandwich
- A handful of dried fruit and nuts
- A few rice cakes with Jam and cottage cheese
- A meal replacement (protein/carbohydrate) shake.

POST-WORKOUT MEALS

- Pasta with tomato pasta sauce, grilled fish and salad
- Jacket potato, chicken breast baked in foil, broccoli and carrots
- Bean and vegetable hotpot with wholegrain bread
- Pitta bread, falafel and salad
- Rice with grilled turkey and steamed vegetables

- Lasagne or vegetable lasagne with salad
- Fish pie with cabbage and cauliflower
- Chilli or vegetarian chilli with rice and a green vegetable
- Dahl (lentils) with rice and vegetables
- Chicken curry with rice and vegetables
- Mashed or baked potato with grilled salmon and salad.

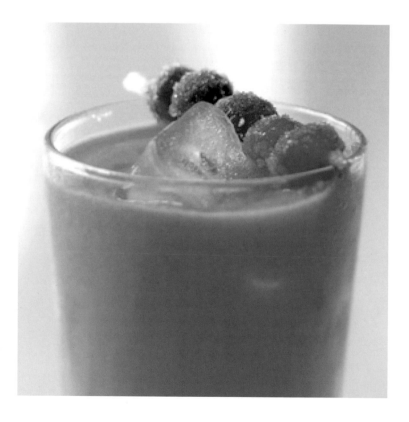

WHAT TO DRINK

You need to replace the fluid you have lost during exercise as soon as possible. Failure to do so can leave you feeling listless and with a headache.

As a rule of thumb, you need to drink 750 ml of water for every $\frac{1}{2}$kg (1 lb) of body weight lost during your workout. Drinking slowly, rather than guzzling the lot in one go, will hydrate you better. Water, diluted juice and sports drinks are all good fluid replacers.

Unless you have been sweating heavily, electrolyte (mineral salts) loss is less critical than water loss. Food eaten in your next normal meal easily replaces electrolytes. But if you have been exercising hard for longer than 1 hour and lost a lot of fluid through sweating, you may need to replace those electrolytes straight away with a sports drink. The sodium in sports drinks helps your body to better retain the fluid.

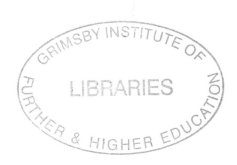

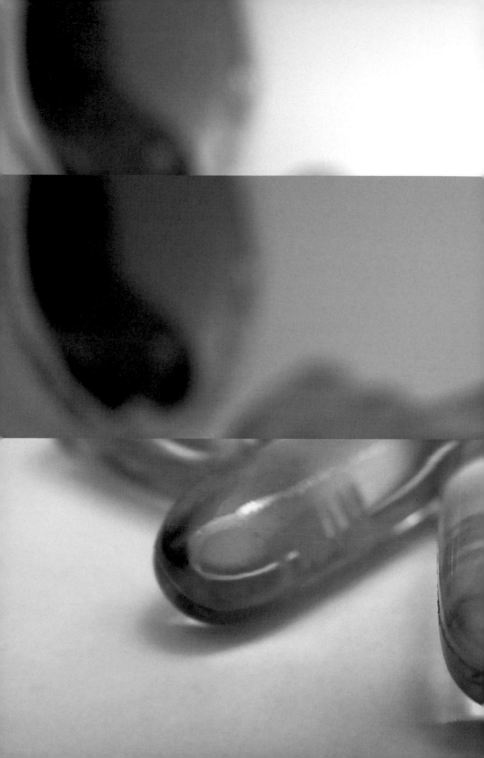

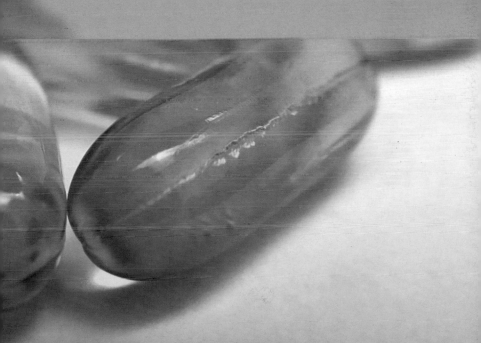

4 SPORTS SUPPLEMENT DIRECTORY

ACETYL L-CARNITINE

See 'Carnitine', page 49.

ALPHA-LIPOIC ACID (ALA)

What is it?

Alpha-lipoic acid (ALA) is produced in the body in small amounts and is also found in red meat. It is a potent antioxidant.

What does it do?

It can help to neutralise damaging free radicals in cells, as well as increase the effects of other antioxidants such as vitamins C and E and glutathione. Studies with animals and diabetics suggest that it may help reduce insulin resistance – acting like insulin itself. Supplements may, therefore, help improve blood sugar control in diabetics.

Do you need it?

First, aim to increase your antioxidant intake by eating plenty of fresh fruit and vegetables, as well as whole grains, nuts and seeds. Antioxidant supplements (*see* Antioxidant supplements, page 39) may help to promote recovery after intense exercise and to reduce cellular damage. ALA is a popular ingredient in certain antioxidant formulations, so taking a single supplement is probably unnecessary.

Are there any side effects?

Diabetics should consult their doctor before taking ALA. It is not recommended for pregnant and breastfeeding women.

ANDROSTENEDIONE ('ANDRO')

What is it?

Androstenedione is a 'pre-hormone', meaning that it is a precursor of both female (oestrogen) hormones and male (testosterone) hormones. It is marketed to increase strength and muscle mass for bodybuilders and strength athletes. It may be sold separately or combined with other pre-hormones (*see* 'Pre-hormones', page 105).

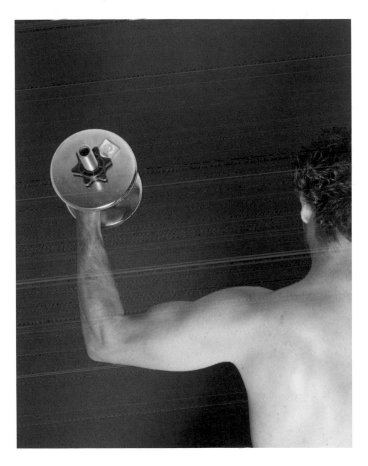

What does it do?

In the body, 'andro' is converted into testosterone. High levels of testosterone can increase muscle strength and size, and enable athletes to exercise more intensely and recover more quickly. However, there is no credible research to back its claims. A study published in the Journal of the American Medical Association in 2000 found that andro supplements failed to elevate testosterone, or increase strength or muscle mass in weight lifters. Although the andro supplements raised androstenedione levels in the blood, there was no effect on muscle mass, either in the short or long term.

Do you need it?

This supplement cannot be recommended because studies have shown that it does not live up to its claims of increasing testosterone levels, enhanced muscle mass and strength. It is also associated with serious side effects (see below). Higher doses than those recommended on supplement labels may result in a failed drugs test for testosterone.

Are there any side effects?

Andro supplements can increase oestrogen levels (which can lead to gynecomastia, male breast development) and decrease HDL (good cholesterol) levels. Reduced HDL carries a greater risk of heart disease. Other side effects include acne, enlarged prostate and water retention.

More about androstenedione

In a study, known as the 'Andro Project', researchers at East Tennessee State University, USA, measured the effects of andro supplements in 50 men aged between 35 and 65 and found no evidence to back up the manufacturer's claims. The men took part in a 12-week weight-training programme and were given either 200 mg androstenedione, 200 mg andro or a placebo (dummy pill). Although testosterone levels increased by 16 per cent after 1 month in those taking the androstenedione, by the end of 12 weeks they went back to normal. That's because their bodies shut down their own production of testosterone. All the men got stronger during the 12-week programme, but there was no difference between those taking the andro supplements and those taking the placebo. What is more, levels of the female hormone oestrogen rose in those using supplements! This could lead to feminisation over a period of time, the opposite of what male strength trainers want to achieve.

ANTIOXIDANT SUPPLEMENTS

What are they?

Antioxidant supplements contain various combinations of anti-oxidant nutrients and plant extracts, including beta-carotene, vitamin C, vitamin E, zinc, magnesium, copper, lycopene (pigment found in tomatoes), selenium, co-enzyme Q10, catechins (found in green tea), methionine (an amino acid) and anthocyanidins (pigments found in purple or red fruit).

What do they do?

Intense exercise generates increased numbers of free radicals. This may deplete the body's antioxidant stores and increase the risk of free radical damage to cells. Left unchecked, free radicals can harm cell membranes, disrupt DNA, destroy enzymes and increase the risk of atherosclerosis and cancer. High levels of free radicals are also associated with post-exercise muscle

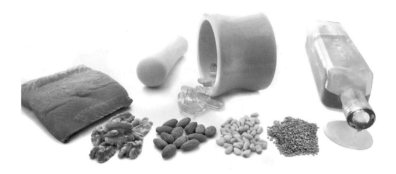

soreness. Supplements of antioxidant nutrients may therefore boost your natural antioxidant defences. Studies have shown that supplements help protect against heart disease, cancer and cataracts, but there is less evidence relating to athletic performance. A 2006 US study showed that antioxidant supplementation improved high-intensity performance in cyclists. On balance, broad spectrum antioxidant supplements (rather than single antioxidants such as vitamin C) help promote recovery after intense exercise and reduce post-exercise muscle soreness.

Do you need them?

Antioxidant supplements may help speed recovery after intense exercise, but should not be a substitute for a healthy diet. Antioxidants – whether from food or supplements – give increased protection from chronic diseases such as heart disease and certain cancers. Aim to eat at least five portions of fruit and vegetables daily – the more intense the colour, the higher the antioxidant content – as well as foods rich in essential fats (such as avocados, oily fish and pure vegetable oils) for their vitamin E content. Scientists at the American Institute for Cancer Research say that eating at least five portions of fruit and vegetables each day can prevent 20 per cent of all cancers. The Department of Health in the UK and the World Health Organisation advise a minimum of 400 g or five portions of fruit and vegetables a day. The average UK intake is just 2.8 portions a day (Food Standards Agency (FSA), 2004).

Are there any side effects?

Side effects are unlikely for antioxidant mixtures. Keep to the recommended doses on the label. Avoid vitamin C intakes over 1000 mg (due to the risk of diarrhoea and stomach upsets) or selenium intakes over 900 micrograms (due to the risk of toxicity). Large doses of carotenoids may turn your skin orange, but this effect is harmless and will gradually go away.

More about antioxidants

Antioxidants are substances that quench free radicals. They include enzymes, vitamins, minerals and phytochemicals.

Exercise causes an increased generation of free radicals, and there is unequivocal evidence that this causes damage to cell membranes. A 2001 study of elite Alpine ski racers found no direct evidence of free radical damage, but measured a drop in the skiers' antioxidant status over a period of intense training. Supplementation may therefore counteract the drop in antioxidant levels in the body and help boost the body's defences against increased free radical attack.

A 2001 Loughborough University study found that daily vitamin C supplementation (200 mg) for 2 weeks reduced muscle soreness and improved recovery following intense exercise. A 2004 US study found that women who took an antioxidant supplement before and after exercise had significantly less damage following weight-training exercise. Sports scientists in South Africa measured enhanced levels of immune

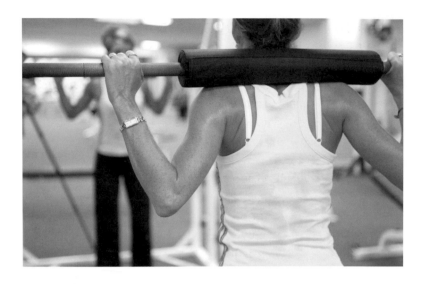

cells (neutrophils) in runners who had taken an antioxidant supplement (vitamin C, vitamin E and beta-carotene) following a strenuous 2-hour run, compared with runners who had been given a placebo.

The EU Recommended Daily Amount for vitamin C is 60 mg and for vitamin E 10 mg. These are levels judged sufficient to support health; they are not optimal amounts for athletic performance or heart disease prevention. A number of scientists believe the UK and US recommended intakes are too low. In *The Ergogenics Edge*, Professor Mel Williams, of the Department of Exercise Science, Physical Education and Recreation at Old Dominion University, Virginia, US, advises 500–1000 mg vitamin C, 250–500 mg vitamin E and 50–100 mg selenium.

BRANCHED-CHAIN AMINO ACID (BCAA) SUPPLEMENTS

What are they?

The BCAAs consist of the three amino acids that have a branched molecular configuration: valine, leucine and isoleucine. They are found in meat, fish, eggs, milk and other protein sources.

What do they do?

BCAAs may be used as a fuel source during endurance exercise, particularly when muscle glycogen is depleted. Supplements may therefore have a protein-sparing effect. Studies at the University of Guelph, Ontario, Canada, in 1994 suggest that taking BCAA supplements during and after exercise can reduce muscle break-down. A study at the University of Tasmania, Australia, concluded that BCAA may help promote faster recovery.

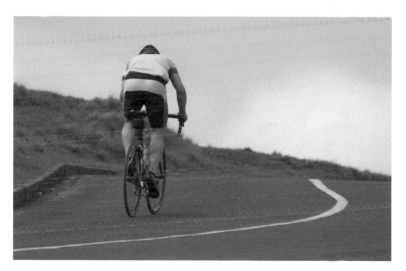

However, it is not clear whether chronic BCAA supplementation benefits performance. Studies with long-distance cyclists at the University of Virginia, US, found that supplements taken before and during a 100 km bike performance test did not improve endurance compared with taking a carbohydrate drink. Studies with strength or power athletes do not exist, but one study with ski mountaineers found that BCAAs had no effect on muscle mass or strength.

Do you need them?

BCAA supplements have limited benefits. They probably won't improve your endurance, but at doses of 6–15 g (as used in the studies at the University of Virginia) they may help improve your recovery during hard training periods by reducing muscle protein breakdown and post-exercise injuries. BCAAs are found in good amounts in most protein supplements (especially whey protein supplements) and meal replacement products, so it is probably not worth taking them if you already use one of these products.

Are there any side effects?

BCAAs are relatively safe as they are normally found in protein in the diet. Excessive intake may reduce the absorption of other amino acids into the body.

CAFFEINE

What is it?

Caffeine is classed as a pharmaceutical compound (drug) rather than a nutrient, but caffeine is often considered a nutritional supplement because it is found in many everyday foods and drinks such as coffee, black and green tea, cola, chocolate, certain

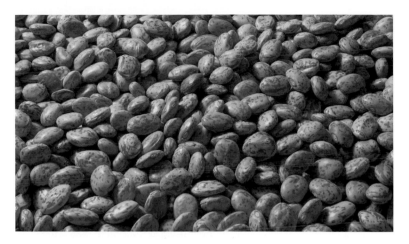

energy and sports drinks and certain energy gels. However, the caffeine content of coffee can vary enormously depending how you make it.

HOW MUCH CAFFEINE?

Product	Caffeine content, mg/cup
Instant coffee	60 mg
Espresso	45–100 mg
Cafetiere/filter	60–120 mg
Tea	40 mg
Green tea	40 mg
Energy drinks	100 mg
Cola	40 mg
Energy gel (1 sachet)	25 mg
Dark chocolate (50 g)	40 mg
Milk chocolate (50 g)	12 mg

What does it do?

Caffeine acts on the central nervous system, increasing alertness and concentration, which could be considered advantageous in many sports. It stimulates adrenaline release, which raises fatty acid levels in the bloodstream. During exercise, your muscles will be able to use more fatty acids for fuel, which conserves valuable glycogen. This means that you can work out longer without feeling tired.

Caffeine can also improve muscle contraction by releasing calcium from its storage sites in muscle cells.

There is a huge amount of research evidence showing that caffeine improves performance in endurance activities. However, the benefits for short-term, high-intensity activities, such as sprinting, are less clear with roughly half the studies suggesting an improvement in performance; half suggesting no benefit. An analysis of 40 caffeine studies by researchers at the University of Luton, UK, showed that caffeine can improve endurance by an average of 12 per cent. Another study with swimmers showed a 23-second improvement in a 21-minute swim. Researchers at RMIT University, Victoria, Australia, found that caffeine improved performance by 4–6 seconds in competitive rowers during a 2000 m row.

Do you need it?

Drinking two cups of coffee or a caffeinated energy drink about an hour before exercise may encourage your muscles to burn more fat and thus help you keep going for longer. In 2002, Canadian researchers found that taking more than two cups of coffee has no additional effect. Australian researchers have found that 1.5 mg/kg (105 mg for a 70 kg athlete) taken in divided doses (e.g. four caffeine-containing energy gels over 2 hours) throughout an intense workout benefits performance in serious athletes. To make the most of its benefits, drink coffee with no or only a small amount of (low fat) milk, because milk slows down caffeine absorption.

Are there any side effects?

Some people are more susceptible to side effects than others. Side effects include anxiety, trembling and sleeplessness. Caffeine also increases your heart rate and breathing rate. If you are sensitive to caffeine, it is best to avoid it.

Scientific research shows, on balance, no link between long-term caffeine use and health problems such as hypertension and bone mineral loss. The connection between raised cholesterol levels and heavy coffee consumption is now known to be caused by certain fats in coffee, which are more pronounced in boiled coffee than instant or filter coffee.

Although caffeine is a diuretic, a daily intake of less than 300 mg results in no larger urine output than water. At this level, caffeine is considered safe and unlikely to have any detrimental effect on performance or health. Taking caffeine regularly (e.g. drinking coffee) builds up your caffeine tolerance so you experience smaller diuretic effects.

More about caffeine

Contrary to popular belief, caffeine taken immediately before exercise does not promote dehydration. In a study at Ohio State University, USA, in 1997, six cyclists consumed a sports drink both with and without caffeine over a 3-hour cycle ride. Researchers found that there was no difference in performance or urine volume during exercise. There was only an increase in urine output at rest.

In another study, when 18 healthy men consumed 1.75 l of three different fluids at rest, the caffeine-containing drink did not change their hydration status.

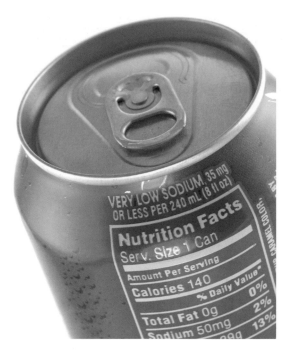

Researchers at the University of Maastricht, the Netherlands, found that cyclists were able to rehydrate after a long cycle equally well with water or a caffeine-containing cola drink. A 2005 study at the University of Connecticut, USA, found that both caffeine-containing cola and caffeine-free cola maintained hydration in athletes (during the non-exercise periods) over three successive days of training. The athletes drank water during training sessions, but they rehydrated with either caffeinated or caffeine-free drinks. A further study by the same researchers confirmed that moderate caffeine intakes (up to 452 mg caffeine per kg body weight per day) did not increase urine output compared with a placebo and concluded that caffeine does not cause a fluid electrolyte balance in the body.

CAFFEINE FOR COMPETITION

If you're looking for that extra competitive edge, come off caffeine for a few days or significantly decrease your intake prior to a competition. This reduces your tolerance so that when you reintroduce caffeine to your system, you'll receive a greater response again. Just before the competition, take approximately 150–200 mg of caffeine from drinks, such as coffee (1–2 strong cups) or an energy/sports drink (1–2 cans).

CARNITINE

What is it?

L-carnitine is a non-essential amino acid made in the liver from the amino acids lysine and methionine. It is essential for energy production and for fat metabolism. It can also be found in meat and dairy products. Most brands of supplements are sold as acetyl-L-carnitine, which is a better-absorbed form of L-carnitine.

What does it do?

The main role of L-carnitine is to transport fatty acids into the mitochondria – the powerhouses of cells – where they are used for energy. The idea of supplementation is to increase levels of carnitine and help the body burn more fat. In theory, this would be advantageous for weight control as well as for endurance. A greater reliance on fat for energy during exercise would help spare muscle glycogen and delay fatigue. However, despite the marketing hype, there is little scientific evidence to support these theories. While initial studies in the 1980s suggested a performance benefit, more recent studies have failed to show that supplements increase fat burning or improve endurance performance.

Do you need it?

As there is little evidence to support the claims made for acetyl-L-carnitine, it cannot be recommended as a performance-boosting supplement to athletes.

Are there any side effects?

No adverse effects have been reported.

CASEIN

What is it?

Casein is a milk protein. It is available as calcium caseinate (a powder which can be mixed with milk or water to make a shake), but it is also a major ingredient in protein supplements and meal replacement products.

What does it do?

Casein comprises larger protein molecules, which are digested and absorbed more slowly than whey. It contains high levels of essential amino acids (and hence a high biological value). Casein is an especially rich source of the immunity-boosting muscle-sparing amino acid glutamine – approximately 20 per cent higher than whey, egg or soy sources (see 'Glutamine', page 78). Casein digests more slowly than whey and for this reason is sometimes considered a 'time-released' protein.

Do you need it?

Casein is less expensive than other protein supplements. Consider adding it to your diet if you have particularly high protein needs and/or during periods of intense training. Strength athletes, such as bodybuilders and power lifters, require 1.4 to 1.8 g per kg body weight per day, which may be difficult to obtain

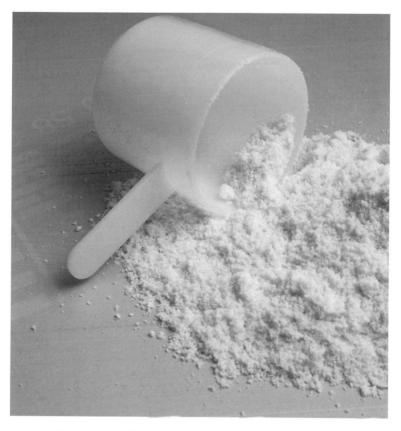

solely from food sources. Adding a protein supplement such as casein can help make up any dietary shortfall, and reduce protein breakdown during intense training.

Are there any side effects?
High intakes are unlikely to have any harmful effect in healthy people, but neither do they provide an advantage in terms of strength or muscle mass.

COLOSTRUM

What is it?

Colostrum is the 'pre-milk' produced from the mother's mammary glands prior to producing milk. Colostrum for supplements is derived from cow's milk and is sometimes called bovine colostrum.

What does it do?

Bovine colostrum contains whey protein, casein and various immune factors (immunoglobulins or antibodies) and growth factors, which are thought to be the same as those in human milk. The theory behind the supplement is that if this formula allows newborn babies to thrive and grow at a rapid rate, it will produce similar benefits in athletes, i.e. improved performance and muscle growth. Preliminary research has produced mixed results with rowers, cyclists and runners. Some studies

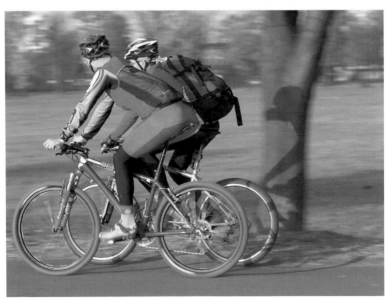

have suggested that it may help build muscle and boost performance, but more research is needed to confirm the benefits.

Do you need it?

Scientists have debated the value of colostrum supplements for many years. Most studies suggest that it is useful for promoting immune function and maintaining a healthy digestive system, but (subject to more research) it may also help improve exercise performance, muscle growth and recovery.

Are there any side effects?

It is not recommended for pregnant or lactating women.

CONJUGATED LINOLEIC ACID (CLA)

What is it?

CLA is an unsaturated fatty acid (in fact, it is a mixture of linoleic acid isomers) found naturally in small amounts in full fat milk, meat and cheese. Supplements are made from sunflower and safflower oils.

What does it do?

It is sold as a fat loss supplement. Studies suggest that it may help reduce fat storage and increase fat burning. Norwegian researchers observed a 20 per cent reduction in body fat after volunteers took 3 g per day for 3 months.

It is thought that CLA works by stimulating hormone-sensitive lipase (which releases fat from fat cells) and suppressing lipo-protein lipase (which transports fat into fat cells).

When combined with resistance training, CLA may also increase muscle mass and strength. University of Memphis researchers found that, compared with a placebo, CLA improved strength in experienced weight lifters. A study of novice bodybuilders at Kent State University, Ohio, USA, found that six weeks of supplementation resulted in increased arm circumference, total muscle mass and overall strength, compared with a placebo group.

Do you need it?
CLA may help reduce your body fat while maintaining or increasing muscle mass. Most researchers recommend 2–5 g per day (divided into three doses).

Are there any side effects?
None have been reported to date.

CREATINE
What is it?
Creatine is a protein that is made naturally in the body from three amino acids (arginine, glycine and methionine), but can also be found in meat and fish or taken in higher doses as a supplement. It is available as a single supplement, and is an ingredient in 'all-in-one' supplements and supplement 'stacks'.

What does it do?
Creatine combines with phosphorus to form phosphocreatine (PC) in your muscle cells. This is an energy-rich compound that fuels your muscles during high-intensity activities, such as lifting weights or sprinting. Boosting PC levels with supplements (typically around 20 per cent) enables you to sustain all-out effort longer than usual, and recover faster between sets, resulting in greater strength and improved ability to do repeated sets. This may lead to faster gains in strength and lean body mass.

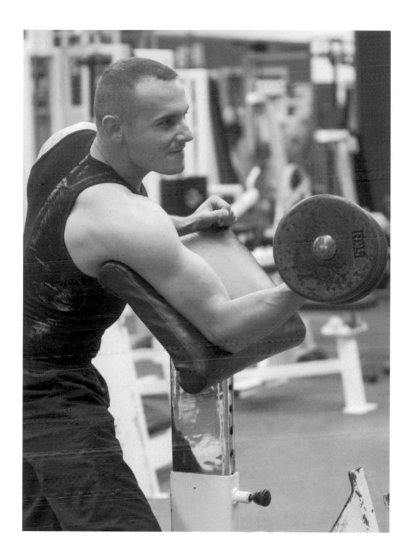

Studies have shown that creatine supplements can improve performance in high-intensity activities (e.g. performing more reps or sets), speed recovery between sets, as well as increase total and lean body weight.

Do you need it?

If you train with weights; sprint or do any sport that includes repeated high-intensity movements, such as sprints, jumps or throws (as in, say, rugby and football), creatine supplements may help increase your performance, strength and muscle mass. Researchers at the Australian Institute of Sport found that creatine improved sprint times and agility-run times in football players. But creatine may not work for everyone – several studies have found that creatine made no difference to performance. And don't bother with creatine if you're an endurance athlete – it does not increase endurance performance.

Are there any side effects?

The main side effect is weight gain. This is due partly to extra water in the muscle cells and partly to increased muscle tissue. While this is desirable for bodybuilders and people who work out with weights, it could be disadvantageous in sports where

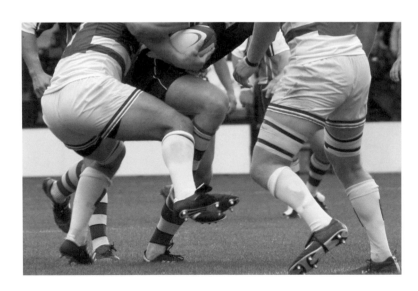

there is a critical ratio of body weight and speed (e.g. running) or in weight-category sports. Some people find they get water retention, particularly during the loading phase. Other reported side effects include cramps and stomach discomfort, which may be due to dehydration rather than creatine. As larger-than-normal amounts of creatine need to be processed by the kidneys, there is a theoretical long-term risk of kidney damage. While short-term and low-dose creatine supplementation appears to be safe, the effects of long-term and/or high-dose creatine supplementation, alone or in combination with other supplements, remain unknown.

More about creatine
■ Performance
Hundreds of studies have measured the effects of creatine supplements on anaerobic performance. Just over half of these report a positive effect on performance; the remainder show no real effect. Studies reviewed in the Journal of Strength and Conditioning Research in 1996 found supplements improved strength (1 rep-max), the number of repetitions performed to fatigue, and the ability to perform repeated sprints.

The vast majority of studies show that short-term creatine supplementation increases body mass. Professor Kreider of the University of Memphis, Tennessee, USA, estimates athletes can gain up to 1.5 kg during the first week of a loading dose and up to 4.5 kg after 6 weeks. Dozens of studies show significant increases in lean mass and total mass, typically between 1 and 3 per cent lean body weight (approx. 0.8–3 kg) after a 5-day loading dose, compared with controls. The observed gains in weight are due partly to an increase in body water content and partly to muscle synthesis. When muscle cell creatine concentration goes up, water is drawn into the cell – rather like filling a balloon – an effect that boosts the thickness of muscle fibres by around 15 per cent. The water content of muscle fibres stretches the cells' outer sheaths – a mechanical force that can trigger growth. This may stimulate protein synthesis and may also result in increased lean tissue.

Creatine may also help muscle cells to grow by increasing levels of insulin-like growth factor-1 (IGF-1), a hormone crucial for muscle growth in muscle cells. In studies at the University of Memphis, athletes taking creatine gained more body mass than those taking the placebo. If creatine improves the quality of resistance training over time, this would lead to faster gains in mass, strength and power.

There is less evidence to show that the use of creatine is beneficial to endurance athletes. This is probably due to the fact that the PC energy system is less important during endurance activities. However, one study at Louisiana State University, Kentucky, USA, suggests creatine supplements may be able to boost athletes' lactate threshold and, therefore, prove beneficial for certain aerobic-based sports.

■ Different forms of creatine supplements
Creatine monohydrate is the most widely available form of creatine. It comprises a molecule of creatine with a molecule of water attached to it, so it is very stable. Other forms of creatine such as creatine alpha keto-glutarate, creatine gluconate, creatine ethyl ester, creatine methyl ester, tricreatine orotate and creatine citrate, claim that they are better absorbed than creatine monohydrate, pass across cell membranes more easily and result in greater uptake by the muscles. However, there is no evidence that these alternative forms of creatine produce higher levels of phosphocreatine in the muscle cells or result in greater increases

in performance or muscle mass. All ultimately produce a similar result.

■ Creatine know-how

The most popular dosage is a 5-day creatine loading phase: 20–25 g daily for 5–7 days, followed by a maintenance dose of 2–5 g daily. While this method gives quick results, it is more likely to produce side effects such as water retention. Also, the body has to work harder to process the excess creatine, as less than 1 per cent of the dose ends up in the muscles. The rest is excreted in the urine. More recent research has shown that lower daily doses of 3–7 g (divided into four equal doses) for 30 days gives similar performance results, but with less water retention. Canadian researchers found that 7 g daily produces significant increases in workout intensity, power output and muscle size in 21 days. On average, the volunteers gained 2.2 kg of lean body weight.

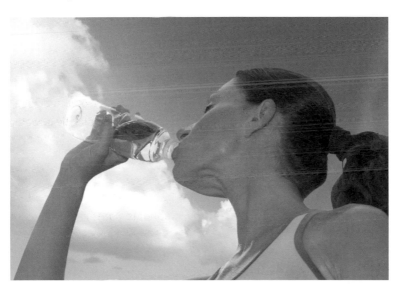

Drink plenty of water – around 2 l daily – to ensure cells have enough to draw in and to expand.

Researchers recommend taking creatine with carbohydrate because the insulin spike produced by the carbohydrates drives more creatine into the muscles. The exact amount of carbohydrates is debatable, but most studies have used between 30 and 90 g. Taking creatine with your normal meals is a cheaper and equally effective option to buying more expensive creatine-carbohydrate products.

Creatine uptake may be greater immediately after exercise, so adding creatine to the post-exercise meal will help to boost muscle creatine levels. Alpha-lipoic acid (an antioxidant) and whey protein also appear to increase creatine uptake.

WILL I LOSE STRENGTH IF I STOP TAKING CREATINE SUPPLEMENTS?

When you stop taking supplements, muscle creatine levels will drop back to normal levels over a period of 4 weeks. During supplementation your body's own synthesis of creatine is depressed, but this is reversible. Certainly, fears that your body permanently shuts down normal creatine manufacture are unfounded. You may experience weight loss, and there are anecdotal reports about athletes experiencing small reductions in strength and power, although not back to pre-supplementation levels.

It has been proposed that creatine is best taken in cycles, such as 3–5 months followed by a 1-month break.

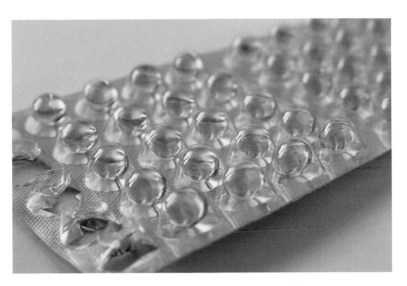

DHEA (DEHYDROEPIANDROSTERONE)

What is it?

DHEA is an androgenic hormone produced by the adrenal glands. Sometimes called 'the mother of all steroid hormones', it is converted in the body into several other hormones such as testosterone, oestrogen and progesterone.

DHEA levels rise during puberty, peak around the age of 30, and then drop off dramatically in both men and women, as they get older. By age 80 you produce only 5 per cent of the DHEA you produced at age 30.

It is often promoted as a 'fountain of youth' supplement. DHEA is marketed for building muscle mass, increasing strength, decreasing body fat and increasing libido.

What does it do?

The theory behind supplement action is that DHEA boosts testosterone levels, which in turn increase lean muscle mass and libido, and reduces body fat.

Do you need it?

In 1996, the Food and Drug Administration (FDA) banned DHEA from the over-the-counter market, because there was no support for the health claims made for it and there were safety concerns. However, it can still be bought from websites. You should be aware that samples may not be properly labelled – one study found big differences between the amounts of DHEA stated on the label and the amounts actually present in the product. Only 44 per cent contained what the label claimed; some contained only trace amounts. It should not be taken by anyone competing in drug-tested sports – DHEA may cause testosterone levels to exceed the IOC limits for testosterone doping.

Are there any side effects?

Since DHEA is converted to testosterone, long-term use may cause potentially fatal liver cysts and liver cancer, increased risk of prostate and breast cancers, blood clotting, steroid-like side effects (increased facial hair, acne, mood swings), raised cholesterol and heart attacks. Long-term usage in women leads to the development of more masculine characteristics such as a deeper voice, excessive body hair and acne. In men, DHEA use can lead to gynecomastia (male breast development) due to increased oestrogen levels.

ENERGY BARS

What are they?

Energy bars are essentially a concentrated carbohydrate source. The main ingredients include maltodextrin (a carbohydrate derived from corn starch), corn syrup, sugars (e.g. fructose, glucose, sucrose), and sometimes also dried fruit or cereal (e.g. rice flour, oat flakes). Most provide around 200 calories and 50 g of carbohydrate per bar with very little protein or fat. Some

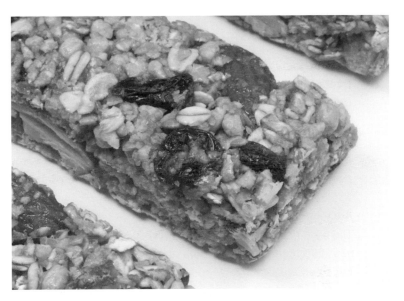

brands may also contain added vitamins and minerals, caffeine, glutamine, taurine or chromium.

What do they do?

Energy bars provide a convenient energy and carbohydrate source. According to a University of Sydney study, consuming solid carbohydrates such as energy bars (with water) before, during or after intense exercise (lasting one hour or longer) is just as effective as consuming liquid carbohydrates (such as sports drinks). Both forms improve endurance because they provide a sustained release of energy. Another Australian study with cyclists compared an energy bar (plus water) with a sports drink during exercise. Both boosted blood sugar levels and endurance. Researchers at Cornell University, New York, USA, found that solid and liquid carbohydrates were, again, equally effective in promoting glycogen re-fuelling after intense and prolonged exercise.

Do you need them?

If you exercise for one hour or longer, energy bars can help maintain your blood sugar levels and postpone fatigue. They are also convenient post-exercise snacks for re-fuelling glycogen stores. Make sure that you have your bar with enough water (at least 250 ml) to replace fluids lost in sweat as well as to digest the bar. Check the label, as some brands are loaded with pure sugar (glucose, corn syrup, fructose, etc.), which produces a surge in blood sugar and insulin. The box below will help you choose the right bar.

Are there any side effects?

The main risk is weight gain if you consume more calories than you burn during exercise. Bars are calorie-dense and come in large portions.

HOW TO CHOOSE THE RIGHT ENERGY BAR

- Check portion sizes – consume no more than 30 g carbs per hour of exercise.
- Check that the bar contains no more than 5 g of fat per 200 calories. Fat slows digestion, which can make you feel heavy and nauseous during exercise.
- Some of the bars are sticky and may adhere to your teeth. Make sure you rinse your mouth well with water after eating a bar. Better still, brush your teeth after your workout.
- For a cheaper alternative, try cereal bars or breakfast bars (opt for varieties that do not contain hydrogenated fats).

ENERGY DRINKS (SEE ALSO 'SPORTS DRINKS', PAGE 107)

What are they?

The principle ingredients of energy drinks are carbohydrate (in the form of sucrose, glucose, fructose and maltodextrin) and

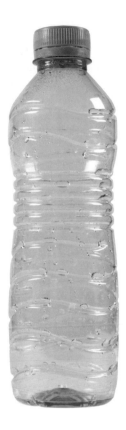

water. They contain higher concentrations of carbohydrate than most sports drinks – typically between 8 and 20 g per 100 ml. Many products also contain electrolytes (such as sodium and potassium), caffeine, protein, herbs, amino acids, vitamins and other substances.

What do they do?
The objective is to deliver extra carbs – useful for boosting endurance during intense exercise lasting more than 60 minutes. Energy drinks can help maintain normal blood glucose levels,

replenish fluid losses and delay fatigue. Energy drinks with electrolytes help replace the salts lost in sweat and help to reduce cramping. Drinks containing a high proportion of maltodextrin are usually easier to digest and provide a steadier release of energy than drinks containing mostly simple sugars, e.g. sucrose, glucose or fructose.

The caffeine may help increase endurance as it raises blood levels of fatty acids, thus sparing muscle glycogen and delaying fatigue. However, any herbal ingredients in energy drinks are usually present in too low a concentration to have a positive health or performance benefit. Energy drinks with a high maltodextrin content are usually isotonic (containing the same concentration of particles as body fluids), which means they can be absorbed faster than water. Drinks with a high content of simple sugars are usually hypertonic (contain a higher concentration of particles than body fluids) and will be absorbed more slowly than water.

Do you need them?

You may benefit from an energy drink if you train hard for more than 60 minutes. Aim for 300–450 ml per hour of an energy drink containing 12 g carbohydrate per 100 ml. Sip around 100 ml every 15 minutes. If you're still thirsty afterwards, or failed to drink during the session, another 200–400 ml may be required. However, you should avoid hypertonic energy drinks (containing more than 8 g sugars per 100 ml) as they can impede rehydration and cause side effects (*see* page 67).

Energy drinks with a little protein may be worth a try. Research suggests that a little protein in a carbohydrate drink can improve performance during exercise.

Recovery energy drinks usually contain around 70 per cent carbohydrate and 30 per cent protein and are designed for rapid replenishment of glycogen stores and kick-starting muscle repair immediately after exercise.

Are there any side effects?
Hypertonic drinks before, during or after exercise may cause gastrointestinal problems, e.g. discomfort, bloating, vomiting and diarrhoea. Drinks with high fructose content can have a laxative effect.

ENERGY GELS
What are they?
Energy gels come in small squeezy sachets and have a jelly-like texture. They consist of simple sugars (such as fructose and glucose) and maltodextrin (a carbohydrate derived from corn starch, consisting of 4–20 glucose units). They may also contain sodium, potassium and, sometimes, caffeine. Most contain between 18 and 25 g of carbohydrate per sachet.

What do they do?
Gels provide a concentrated source of calories and carbohydrate and are designed to be consumed during endurance exercise. Studies show that consuming 30–60 g of carbohydrate per hour during prolonged exercise delays fatigue and improves endurance. This translates into 1–2 sachets per hour. One study showed that gels have a similar effect on blood sugar levels and performance as sports drinks.

Do you need them?
Energy gels provide a convenient way of consuming carbohydrate during intense endurance exercise lasting longer than an hour. But you need to drink around 350 ml of water with each 25 g carb gel to dilute it to a 7 per cent carb solution in your

stomach. Try half a gel with 175 ml (six big gulps) every 15–30 minutes. On the downside, some people dislike their texture, sweetness and intensity of flavour – it's really down to personal preference – and they don't do away with the need for carrying a water bottle with you.

Are there any side effects?

Energy gels don't hydrate you, so you must drink plenty of water with them. If you don't drink enough, you'll end up with gelatinous goo in your stomach. This drags water from your bloodstream into your stomach, increasing the risk of dehydration.

EPHEDRINE/EPHEDRA

See 'Ma Huang', page 88.

EPIGALLOCATECHIN GALLATE (EGCG)

See 'Green tea extract', page 81.

'FAT BURNERS' OR THERMOGENIC PRODUCTS

What are they?

Fat-burning or 'diet' pills claim to speed your metabolism and shed body fat. The main ingredient is ephedrine, or ephedra, a stimulant substance derived from the Chinese herb, ma huang (*see* 'Ma huang', page 88). It is often combined with caffeine and aspirin. Endurance and strength athletes commonly take them to increase workout intensity and duration and to help with weight loss.

Ephedrine is also used at low concentrations in cold and flu remedies (pseudo ephedrine).

What do they do?

Athletes use fat burners because they increase thermogenesis (calorie burning) and metabolic rate. They produce a 'speed-like' effect, making you feel more alert, motivated and confident; they also increase your heart rate and blood pressure. When ephedrine and caffeine are taken together they appear to boost each other's effects. Aspirin is also sometimes added as it may prolong the stimulant activity of the other two. No one knows the precise action, but it is thought that when you take fat burners you temporarily supercharge the nervous system, causing an increase in heat production (or thermogenesis) and release of stored fat. Studies have shown that these supplements do indeed enhance fat loss when taken with a low-calorie diet but this effect decreases over time. The problem is that they can also cause harmful side effects (*see* below).

Do you need them?

These are addictive drugs, and I would strongly recommend avoiding any fat-burner containing ephedrine (or ma huang) because of the significant health risks. The International Olympic Committee (IOC) bans ephedrine. Exercise and good nutrition are the safest methods for burning fat.

Are there any side effects?

Up to 25 mg in one dose is considered safe in cold remedies; higher doses would be needed to produce a stimulant effect. The doses necessary to cause a fat-burning effect are quite high and are associated with a number of risky side effects, including an increased and irregular heartbeat, a rise in blood pressure, insomnia, anxiety, nausea, irritability, dizziness, and other symptoms of nervousness (or being 'hyper'). More severe consequences of high doses, such as heart attack, stroke and death, have been reported in the medical press. Taking the ephedrine-caffeine-aspirin stack increases the chances of side effects even at low doses. In conclusion, the risks far outweigh any potential benefits.

FAT BURNERS (EPHEDRINE-FREE)

What are they?

Certain fat-burning and weight loss supplements claim to mimic the effects of ephedrine, boost the metabolism and enhance fat loss, but without harmful side effects. The main ingredients in these products include citrus aurantium (synephrine or bitter orange extract); green tea extract and Coleus forskohlii extract (a herb, similar to mint).

What do they do?

Citrus aurantium is a weak stimulant, chemically similar to ephedrine and caffeine. It contains a compound called synephrine, which, according to manufacturers reduces appetite, increases the metabolic rate and promotes fat burning. However, despite the hype, there is no sound scientific evidence to back up the weight loss claims.

The active constituents in **green tea** are a family of polyphenols called catechins (the main type is epigallocatechin gallate, EGCG) and flavanols, which possess potent antioxidant activity. Apart from the clear benefits of green tea as an antioxidant, initial research suggests that it may also stimulate thermogenesis, increasing calorie expenditure, and promoting fat burning and weight loss.

The theory behind **Coleus forskohlii** as a dietary supplement is that its content of forskolin can be used to stimulate adenyl cyclase activity, which will increase cAMP levels in the fat cell, which will in turn activate another enzyme (hormone sensitive lipase) to start breaking down fat stores. But there are no published trials showing that Coleus forskohlii extract promotes weight loss.

Do you need them?

The research on ephedrine-free fat burners is not robust, and any fat burning boost they provide would be relatively small or none. The doses used in some brands may be too small to provide a measurable effect. A careful calorie intake and exercise are likely to produce better weight-loss results in the long term. The only positive data is for green tea, but you would need to drink at least six cups daily (equivalent to 100–300 mg EGCG) to achieve a significant fat-burning effect.

Are there any side effects?

While the herbal alternatives to ephedrine are generally safer, you may get side effects with high doses. Citrus aurantium can increase blood pressure as much, if not more, than ephedrine. High doses of forskolin may cause heart disturbances.

FISH OIL

What is it?

Fish oil is a concentrated source of omega-3 fatty acids, in particular the long-chain fatty acids eicosapentanoic acid (EPA) and docosahexanoic acid (DHA).

What do they do?

Omega-3 fatty acids are needed for making a family of hormones called eicosanoids, which are important for regulating blood flow, blood pressure and the immune response, and protecting against cardiovascular disease. EPA and DHA help reduce the tendency for blood clots forming, which can lead to heart attacks

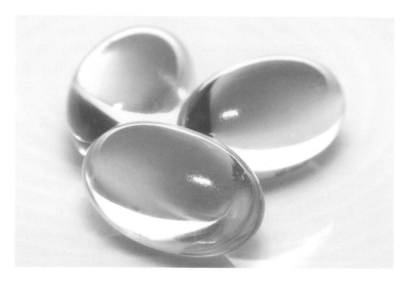

and stroke. They also lower levels of fats in the bloodstream, reduce the risk of irregular heartbeat and help regulate blood pressure. Recent research suggests omega-3s may also help maintain brain function, prevent Alzheimer's disease, treat depression, and help improve behaviour in children with dyslexia, dyspraxia and ADHD.

For regular exercisers, omega-3s increase the delivery of oxygen to muscles, and improve aerobic capacity and endurance. They also help speed recovery, reduce inflammation in the muscles and joints, and reduce joint stiffness.

The long-chain fatty acids are particularly important during pregnancy and lactation to promote brain, nerve and eye development in babies.

Do you need it?

Fish oil supplements are a convenient alternative to oily fish and may be particularly beneficial for regular exercisers. The Food Standards Agency recommends consuming a minimum of one serving (140 g) of oily fish, such as salmon, a week. Most people don't eat enough – the average intake is around 200 mg omega-3s per day, less than half the recommended daily intake of 450 mg. Also, concerns about the levels of mercury and PCBs (a mixture of individual chemicals found in the environment that are related to several health problems) have caused many people to cut back on their fish intake. The good news is that a recent study found no traces of either in more than 40 brands of fish oil supplements.

Consider a fish oil (or other omega-3 rich) supplement if you are pregnant or breastfeeding. Studies show that pregnant women who consume plenty of omega-3s are less likely to give birth to babies with behavioural and learning problems. They are also less likely to suffer postnatal depression. Consuming plenty of omega-3 during breastfeeding increases the omega-3 content of breast milk, which can help promote normal development of the baby's brain, cognitive, nerve and eye tissue.

Are there any side effects?
The main side effect is the fishy taste of the supplement and subsequent fishy breath. However, fruit-flavoured supplements are widely available, which helps to disguise the fish taste.

FLAXSEED OIL
What is it?
Flaxseed oil is one of the richest sources of the short-chain omega-3 fatty acid, alpha-linolenic acid (ALA).

What does it do?
ALA is converted into eicosapentanoic acid (EPA) and docosa-hexanoic acid (DHA) in the body. These fatty acids, which are

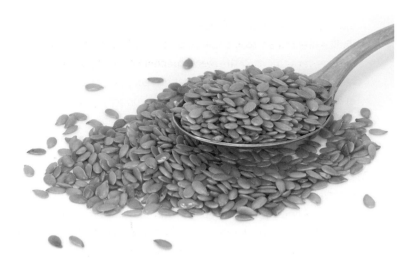

also found in oily fish and fish oils, offer greater cardio protective benefits than the parent ALA, helping reduce blood triglyceride (fat) levels, and heart attack and stroke risk. They also help keep joints supple. For regular exercisers, omega-3s enhance aerobic metabolism, improve oxygen delivery to cells during exercise, help to prevent and heal joint, tendon and ligament strains, and also help reduce inflammation caused by overtraining. But this conversion process is not always efficient – especially if you consume lots of omega-6s (linoleic acid) found in sunflower and most other plant oils – so you need to eat lots of ALA to produce levels of EPA and DHA comparable to those that can be obtained by eating fish.

Do you need it?

Flaxseed oil is particularly beneficial for vegetarians as there are very few plant sources of omega-3s. The Vegetarian Society recommends an ALA intake of 1.5 per cent of energy, or roughly 4 g a day. One tablespoon of flaxseed oil contains approximately 8 g of ALA. Use in salad dressings or drizzled over vegetables. Do not cook with it, as heat alters the chemical composition of the oil and destroys its beneficial properties.

Are there any side effects?
There are no side effects.

GINSENG

What is it?
Ginseng is the collective term for various extracts of the plant Araliaceae, the most important being the ginsenosides. The most common forms of ginseng include Korean (Pana ginseng) and Siberian (Eleutherococcus senticosus).

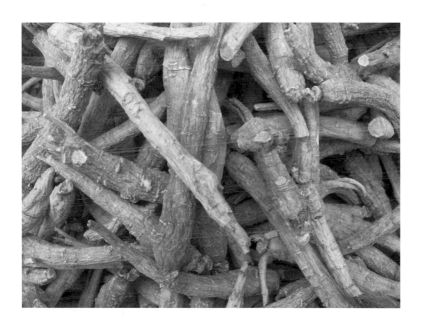

What does it do?

Ginseng is known as an 'adaptogen', which means it helps the body cope better under stress. It has long been used to promote energy and vitality and, more recently, as a performance enhancer for athletes. Manufacturers claim that ginseng enables athletes to train more intensely, increases stamina and improves performance. However, the exact mechanism of its actions in the body is not known. One theory is that it influences the functioning of the adrenal glands and balances the levels of stress hormones such as cortisol. Another is that ginseng acts on the hypothalamus of the brain and sympathetic nervous system to increase blood flow, oxygen delivery and use by muscle cells. Unfortunately, there is a lack of scientific evidence to support ginseng's claims. Studies have failed to show that it increases oxygen uptake, athletic performance or endurance.

Do you need it?

As there is no good evidence to support the claims made for ginseng, it cannot be recommended as a sports supplement.

Are there any side effects?

High doses may cause high blood pressure and insomnia. There is also the risk of contamination – one study found the banned stimulant ephedrine in a sample of ginseng.

GLUCOSAMINE

What is it?

Glucosamine is found naturally in the body. It is an amino sugar and a major component of cartilage, which serves as an important cushioning and shock-absorbing material for the joints. It is also one of the main substances in synovial fluid that lubricates and provides nutrients for joint structures. Supplements are made from crab, lobster and shrimp shells.

What does it do?
Glucosamine supplements may help strengthen tendons, cartilage and ligaments and regenerate damaged cartilage. As the body ages, cartilage loses its elasticity and cushioning properties for joints, which may result in stiffness, immobility and pain. Sports people and regular exercisers sometimes suffer damaged cartilage as a result of years of repetitive motion and overuse of their joints. Glucosamine appears to work by stimulating the cartilage cells to produce proteoglycans (building blocks) that repair joint structures. Thus, supplements can help restore joint function and mobility.

Do you need it?
If you suffer from pain and stiffness in your knees, elbows or shoulders as a result of sports-related overuse, or if you suffer from osteoarthritis, glucosamine supplements may help relieve your symptoms. The recommendation is to take 500 mg with food three times a day. It may take three to eight weeks to produce noticeable results. Glucosamine sulphate has been shown to work more effectively when combined with chondroitin sulphate. This supplement helps stimulate cartilage repair mechanisms and inhibit enzymes that break down cartilage.

Are there any side effects?
Side effects may include stomach discomfort and intestinal gas.

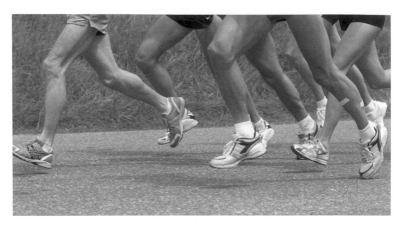

GLUTAMINE

What is it?

Glutamine is a non-essential amino acid found abundantly in the muscle cells and blood. It can be made in the muscle cells from other amino acids (glutamic acid, valine and isoleucine).

What does it do?

Glutamine is needed for cell growth, as well as serving as a fuel for the immune system. During periods of heavy training or stress, blood levels of glutamine fall, weakening your immune system and putting you at risk of infection. Muscle levels of glutamine also fall, which result in a loss of muscle tissue, despite continued training.

Do you need it?

Manufacturers claim that glutamine has a protein-sparing effect during intense training. But the evidence for glutamine is divided. Some studies have shown that taking supplements of glutamine immediately after heavy training or a competitive event, such as a marathon, can help you recover more quickly, reduce muscle soreness, and cut your risk of catching colds and other infections. Others have failed to show any benefits. Canadian researchers found glutamine produced no increase in strength or muscle mass compared with a placebo. Studies have used doses of around 100 mg glutamine per kg of body weight during the 2 hours following a strenuous workout or competition. That's equivalent to a 7 g dose in a 70 kg athlete. But that doesn't mean you will get any benefit. Many protein and meal replacement supplements contain glutamine.

Are there any side effects?
No side effects have been found so far.

More about glutamine
The interest in glutamine stems from the observation that after intense prolonged exercise or during periods of heavy training, blood and muscle glutamine levels tend to fall quite dramatically. There is also a drop in the activity of immune cells, making athletes more susceptible to infection during this time. In other words, without adequate fuel (glutamine), immune cell activity is impaired.

The idea behind glutamine supplementation is that it will prevent the post-exercise drop in glutamine levels and maintain the immune system. Theoretically, glutamine may also prevent the muscle breakdown normally associated with hard training. That's because it helps draw water into the muscle cells, increasing the cell volume. This inhibits enzymes from breaking down muscle proteins and also counteracts the effects of stress hormones, such as cortisol, which are increased after intense exercise.

Studies at Oxford University with marathon runners and ultra-marathon runners have shown that glutamine supplements taken immediately after running and again 2 hours later appeared to lower the risk of infection and boost immune cell activity. Only 19 per cent of those taking glutamine became ill during the week following the run, while 51 per cent of those taking a placebo became ill. However, not all studies have managed to replicate these findings.

While some studies have suggested that supplements may reduce the risk of infection and promote muscle growth, others have failed to show any effect on performance, body composition or muscle breakdown. According to a 2001 study in the European Journal of Applied Physiology, glutamine produces no increase in strength or muscle mass compared with a placebo. After 6 weeks weight training, those taking glutamine achieved the same gains in strength and muscle mass as those taking a placebo.

GLYCEROL

What is it?

Glycerol is a sweet, colourless liquid found naturally in all fats in its glyceride form (it is the 'backbone' of triglycerides). It is used in food products, medicines and skincare products, and is also a popular supplement with endurance athletes.

What does it do?

Glycerol is marketed as a 'hyper-hydration' agent. When taken with plentiful fluids before a prolonged endurance event, it increases hydration in the cells above normal levels. It drags water into both the extra-cellular and intra-cellular fluid and holds it there rather like a sponge. This results in an increase in total body water stores. This can be an advantage during endurance activities, because it allows the tissues to remain hydrated longer. Thus it can help prevent fatigue associated with dehydration and enhance endurance. Studies at the Australian

Institute of Sport found that cyclists retained an extra 600 ml of fluid and improved performance in a time trial by 2.4 per cent following glycerol supplementation.

Do you need it?

It may help improve your performance in prolonged endurance cycling events, particularly under hot or humid conditions. However, the few positive studies with glycerol have been with cyclists. The benefits may not extend to running events, because carrying extra weight can reduce running speed.

Are there any side effects?

A few side effects have been reported, including gastrointestinal upsets and headaches. If you wish to experiment with glycerol, follow the dilution directions on the label carefully and do not consume it undiluted.

GREEN TEA EXTRACT

What is it?

Green tea extract is a popular ingredient in weight loss and fat burning/thermogenics supplements. The active compounds in green tea are a family of polyphenols (catechins) and flavanols, which are potent antioxidants. The main catechins include epicatechin (EC), epigallocatechin (EGC), epicatechin gallate (ECG) and epigallocatechin gallate (EGCG). A number of commercial green tea extracts are standardised to total polyphenol content and/or EGCG content.

What does it do?

EGCG is the most powerful of the catechins, with antioxidant activity about 25–100 times more potent than vitamins C and E. Laboratory studies have shown that it can halt the progression

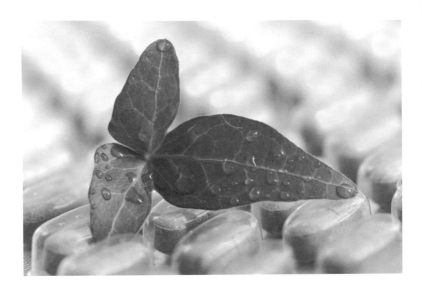

of cancer and epidemiological studies have shown that people with a high intake of polyphenols have a lower risk of cancer and heart disease. Other studies have suggested that green tea extract may also be an effective weight loss supplement. It causes a mild increase in thermogenesis, i.e. calorie burning. This is thought to be due partly to its caffeine content and partly to its catechins and flavanols content. In one study, volunteers were given green tea extract, caffeine or a placebo. The green tea extract increased their daily calorie burn by 80 calories, while the caffeine supplement and placebo resulted in no increase in calorie burning.

Do you need it?
Green tea extract (in doses of 125–500 mg per day) may be worth considering as a weight loss aid in conjunction with an exercise programme. It is often used as an ingredient in weight loss

supplements. However, don't expect miracles – the increased calorie burn is small (80 calories daily).

Are there any side effects?

Green tea is not associated with side effects, but high intakes may lead to restlessness, insomnia and headaches due to the caffeine content. If you are sensitive to caffeine check the ingredients on the supplement label.

GUARANA

What is it?

Guarana comes from the seeds of a South American shrub. Guarana seeds contain twice the caffeine of coffee beans. Supplements contain approximately half the caffeine of coffee.

What does it do?

The main constituent of guarana is caffeine (the same caffeine found in coffee and tea) and typical guarana supplements

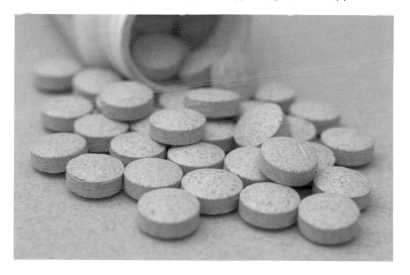

contain 30–50 per cent caffeine. It also contains theobromine and theophylline, also found in coffee and tea. These substances are central nervous system stimulants and can increase the metabolic rate and alertness, and reduce fatigue. Many studies have shown that caffeine can increase endurance and exercise performance.

Guarana is also used as an ingredient in weight loss products marketed to sports people. On its own, it is not a very effective fat burner, although it may help suppress appetite. It is often combined with ma huang (ephedra) and aspirin (see 'Fat burners', page 68) in the 'ECA stack'. Such fat burning supplements suppress appetite and increase daily calorie burn, but as ephedra is associated with a number of serious side effects, such supplements cannot be recommended.

Do you need it?
Guarana may help increase endurance and exercise performance, due to its caffeine content. It is up to you whether you take caffeine in the form of coffee or other caffeine-containing beverages, or guarana – the only consideration is the caffeine concentration. Do not believe marketing claims that guarana is 'more natural' than other forms of caffeine or that it has no side effects.

Are there any side effects?
Guarana may cause the same side effects as caffeine – anxiety, trembling, insomnia, headaches, high blood pressure and heart palpitations.

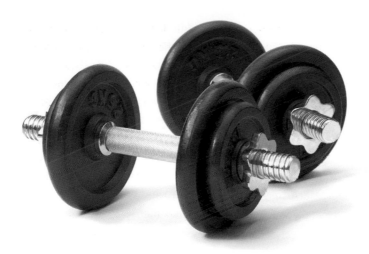

HMB (BETA-HYDROXY BETA-METHYL BUTYRATE)

What is it?

HMB is the by-product of the body's normal breakdown of leucine, an essential amino acid. You can also obtain it from several foods such as grapefruit, alfalfa and catfish.

What does it do?

No one knows exactly how HMB works, but it is thought to be involved with the repair and growth of muscle cells. There is data to show that HMB protects muscle protein from excessive breakdown during intense exercise and accelerates repair after exercise.

Studies at Iowa State University, USA, in the 1990s suggested that HMB may increase strength and muscle mass and reduce muscle damage after resistance exercise. Volunteers experienced average muscle mass gains of 1.2 kg and strength gains of 18 per cent after 3 weeks, compared with a 0.45 kg muscle gain and 8 per cent strength gain from a placebo. But these benefits have not been found in all athletes, particularly with more experienced athletes. One study at the Australian Institute of Sport found that 6 weeks of HMB supplementation had no effect at all on the strength and muscle mass gains in well-conditioned athletes. Researchers at the University of Queensland, Australia, found no beneficial effect on reducing muscle damage or muscle soreness following resistance exercise.

There is some evidence that HMB combined with alpha-ketoisocaproic acid may reduce signs and symptoms of exercise-induced muscle damage in novice weight trainers.

Do you need it?
If you're new to lifting weights, HMB may help boost your strength and build muscle, but probably only for the first 2 months of training. No long-term studies have been carried out to date – it is unlikely to benefit more experienced athletes.

Are there any side effects?
No side effects have yet been found.

INOSINE

What is it?
Inosine is made in the body, mainly in heart and skeletal muscle. It is also found in brewer's yeast, liver and other offal.

What does it do?
It is an essential compound involved in energy metabolism, in particular for transporting oxygen into muscle cells. It increases the formation of 2,3 DPG, a compound in red blood cells that helps to release oxygen to the muscle cells.

Inosine also helps to regenerate the energy compound ATP

mimics the effects of adrenaline and norepinephrine, increasing blood sugar levels. It can also suppress the appetite. Athletes use it because it has a 'speed-like' effect, increasing alertness, motivation and performance. It also increases your heart rate and blood pressure, as well as speeding up your metabolic rate and calorie burn. It is often combined with caffeine and aspirin or salicylates from white willow as a 'fat burner' supplement (see 'Fat burners' page 68) – together they appear to boost each other's effects. Studies have shown that these supplements increase energy expenditure and help speed up fat loss when taken with a low-calorie diet. The problem is that they can also cause harmful side effects (see below).

Do you need it?

Ephedrine is considered a banned substance by the International Olympic Committee (IOC). It is an addictive drug, and I would strongly recommend avoiding ephedrine or ma huang because of the significant health risks.

Are there any side effects?

The doses necessary to cause a fat-burning effect are quite high and are associated with a number of risky side effects, including an increased and irregular heartbeat, a rise in blood pressure, insomnia, anxiety, nausea, irritability and dizziness. More severe consequences, such as heart attack, stroke and death, have been reported in the medical press. Taking the ephedrine-caffeine-aspirin stack increases the chance of side effects, even at low doses. In conclusion, the risks far outweigh any potential benefits.

In 2002, the American Medical Association called for a ban on ephedrine due to concerns over its side effects. Since 1997 the Food and Drug Administration (FDA) in the USA has documented at least 70 deaths and more than 1400 'adverse effects' involving supplements containing ephedrine. These included heart attacks, strokes and seizures.

Ephedrine's risks far outweigh any potential benefits. It is addictive and people can develop a tolerance to it (you need to keep taking more and more to get the same effects). Up to 25 mg in one dose is considered safe in cold remedies; higher doses would be needed to produce a stimulant effect.

MALTODEXTRIN

See Energy bars (page 62); Energy drinks (page 64); Energy gels (page 67), Sports drinks (page 107).

MEAL REPLACEMENT PRODUCTS (MRPs)

What are they?

Meal replacement products (MRPs) are available as powders, ready-to-drink shakes and bars. They contain a mixture of milk proteins (usually whey protein and/or casein), carbohydrate (maltodextrin and/or sugars), vitamins and minerals. Some brands also contain small amounts of unsaturated oils, and other nutrients that claim to boost performance. Weight gain formulas are very similar to MRPs but usually contain more calories in the form of carbohydrates and unsaturated oils to help promote growth.

What do they do?

MRPs provide a nutritionally balanced and convenient alternative to solid food. They are tailored towards aiding muscular growth and recovery.

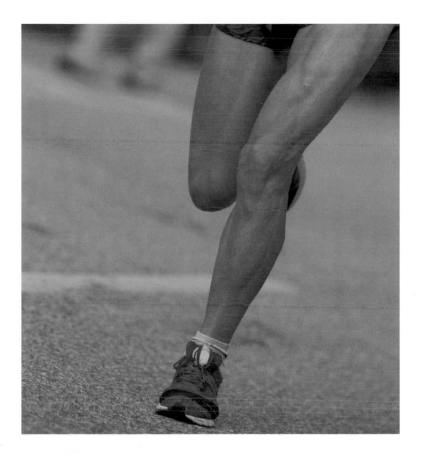

Do you need them?

They will not necessarily improve your performance, but can be a helpful and convenient addition (rather than replacement) to your diet if you struggle to eat enough real food; you need to eat on the move, or you need the extra nutrients they provide.

Are there any side effects?

Side effects are unlikely.

MULTIVITAMIN AND MINERAL SUPPLEMENTS

What are they?

Multivitamin and mineral pills contain a mixture of micronutrients.

What do they do?

Vitamins and minerals are substances needed in tiny amounts to enable your body to work properly and prevent illness. Getting

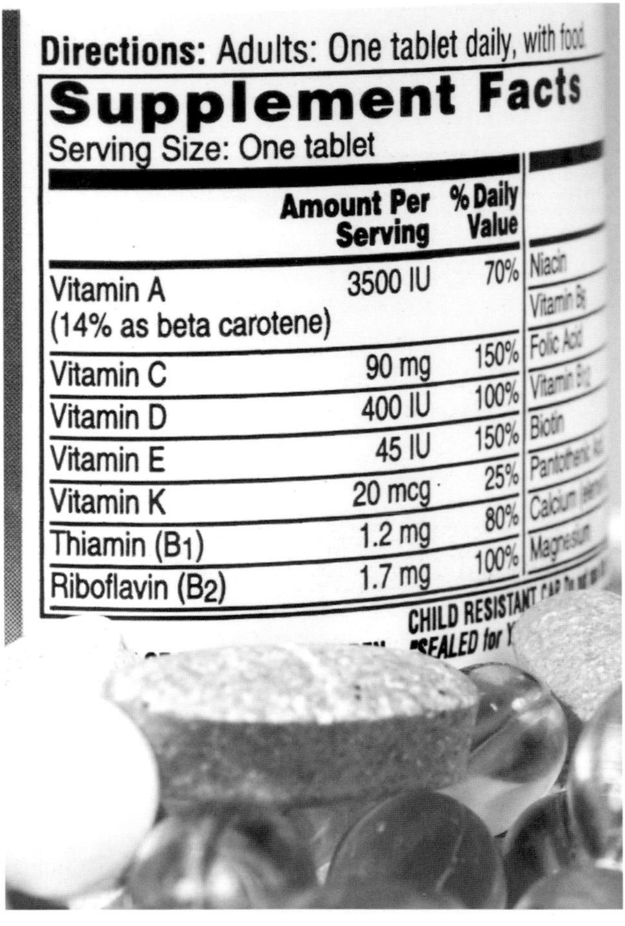

Directions: Adults: One tablet daily, with food.

Supplement Facts

Serving Size: One tablet

	Amount Per Serving	% Daily Value	
Vitamin A (14% as beta carotene)	3500 IU	70%	Niacin
			Vitamin B₆
Vitamin C	90 mg	150%	Folic Acid
Vitamin D	400 IU	100%	Vitamin B₁₂
Vitamin E	45 IU	150%	Biotin
Vitamin K	20 mcg	25%	Pantothenic Acid
Thiamin (B₁)	1.2 mg	80%	Calcium
Riboflavin (B₂)	1.7 mg	100%	Magnesium

CHILD RESISTANT CAP
SEALED for Y

adequate amounts is also important for maximising sports performance. Failure to get enough vitamins and minerals could leave you lacking in energy and susceptible to minor infections and illnesses.

The table on pp. 96–100 summarises the exercise-related functions, best food sources and requirements of 12 key vitamins and minerals.

Supplements can help make up any shortfall in your diet and boost your nutritional status, but there's no evidence that high doses enhance exercise performance.

Do you need them?

Many people would probably benefit from taking a supplement, but popping a pill can't erase the health effects of a poor diet and sedentary lifestyle. Go for real food first and take regular exercise. If you workout intensely several times a week, your requirements for many vitamins and minerals will be greater than the RDAs, so supplements may help you to better meet your needs. A deficiency of any vitamin and mineral will impair your health as well as your performance.

WHAT ARE RDAs?

The Recommended Daily Amounts (RDAs) listed on food and supplement labels are rough estimates of nutrient requirements, set by the EU and designed to cover the needs of the majority of a population. The RDA amounts are designed to prevent deficiency symptoms, allow for a little storage, as well as covering differences in needs from one person to the next. They are not targets; rather they are guides to help you check that you are probably getting enough nutrients.

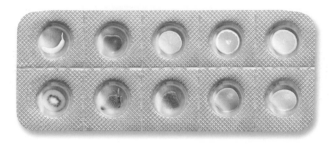

Are there any side effects?

Taking vitamin and mineral supplements is generally harmless but, to safeguard against overdosing, the Food Standards Agency (FSA) has set guidelines on safe upper levels. These include a warning not to exceed 10 mg per day of chromium picolinate. Taking more than 1 g per day of vitamin C may cause an upset stomach, while more than 17 mg per day of iron may cause constipation. Taking more than 10 mg of vitamin B6 over a long period may lead to numbness and persistent pins and needles. High doses of vitamin A should be avoided during pregnancy, as it may result in birth defects. Vitamin D in high doses may cause high blood pressure so, as a general rule, never take more than 10 times the RDA of vitamins A and D, and no more than the RDA for any mineral.

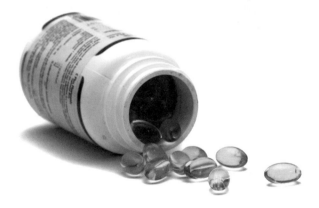

Check the quantities on the label and do not exceed the upper safe levels shown in the table below.

ARE YOU DEFICIENT IN VITAMINS AND MINERALS?

About 12 million people in the UK take vitamin and mineral supplements to prevent or alleviate illnesses. A study published in the Journal of the American Medical Association concluded that most people do not get enough vitamins in their diet to protect themselves properly from diseases such as cancer and heart disease. Researchers at the Harvard Medical School say that most people would benefit from taking a multivitamin, especially if:

■ You are dieting or eating fewer than 1500 calories daily. Restricting your food intake makes it more likely that you are missing out on certain nutrients.

■ You rely mainly on processed or fast foods. These foods are not only high in saturated fat, sugar and salt, but also depleted in vitamins.

■ You regularly skip meals. This means that you are more likely to eat high-calorie snacks that are low in vitamins and minerals.

■ You don't eat the recommended five portions of fruit and vegetables daily. These foods are rich in vitamins, minerals and antioxidants.

■ You have a food intolerance or allergy. It may be harder to get some of the nutrients you need.

■ You are a vegan. It's more difficult (though not impossible) to get enough vitamin B12, calcium and iron from a plant-based diet.

■ You are pregnant. Take a supplement containing 0.4 mg of folic acid and follow the advice of your midwife or doctor.

GUIDE TO VITAMINS AND MINERALS

Vitamin/mineral	How much?*	Why is it needed?
Vitamin A	700 ug (men) 600 ug (women) No SUL FSA recommends 1500 ug max	Helps vision in dim light; promotes healthy skin
Carotenoids	No official RNI 15 mg beta-carotene suggested SUL = 7 mg	Vision in dim light; healthy skin; converts into vitamin A
Thiamin	0.4 mg/1000 kcal No SUL mg FSA recommends 100 mg max	Converts carbohy-drates to energy
Riboflavin	1.3 mg (men) 1.1 mg (women) No SUL mg FSA recommends 40 mg max	Converts carbohy-drates to energy
Niacin	6.6 mg/1000 kcal SUL = 17 mg	Converts carbohy-drates to energy

Why supplements may benefit you	Best food sources	Side effects
Maintain normal vision and healthy skin	Liver, cheese, oily fish, eggs, butter, margarine	Liver and bone damage; can harm unborn babies (avoid during pregnancy)
As antioxidants, may protect against certain cancers and reduce muscle soreness. Exercise increases need for antioxidants.	Intensely coloured fruit and vegetables, e.g. apricots, peppers, tomatoes, mangoes, broccoli	Excessive doses of beta-carotene can cause harmless orange tinge to skin. Reversible.
To process the extra carbohydrate eaten	Wholemeal bread and cereals, pulses, meat	Excess is excreted so toxicity is rare
To process the extra carbohydrate eaten	Milk and dairy products, meat, eggs	Excess is excreted (producing yellow urine!) so toxicity is rare
To process the extra carbohydrate eaten	Meat and offal, nuts, milk and dairy products, eggs, wholegrain cereals	Excess is excreted. High doses may cause hot flushes.

Vitamin C	40 mg SUL = 1000 mg	Healthy connective tissue, bones, teeth, blood vessels, gums and teeth; promotes immune function; helps iron absorption
Vitamin E	No RNI in UK 10 mg in EU SUL = 540 mg	Antioxidant which helps protect against heart disease; promotes normal cell growth and development
Calcium	1000 mg (men) 700 mg (women) SUL = 1500 mg	Builds bone and teeth; blood clotting; nerve and muscle function
Iron	8.7 mg (men) 14.8 mg (women) SUL = 17 mg	Formation of red blood cells; oxygen transport; prevents anaemia
Zinc	9.5 mg (men) 7.0 mg (women) SUL = 25 mg	Healthy immune system; wound healing; skin; cell growth

Exercise increases need for antioxidants; may help reduce free radical damage, protect cell membranes and reduce post-exercise muscle soreness	Fruit and vegetables, e.g. raspberries, blackcurrants, kiwi, oranges, peppers, broccoli, cabbage, tomatoes	Excess is excreted. Doses over 2 g may lead to diarrhoea and excess urine formation. High doses (>2 g) may cause vitamin C to behave as a pro-oxidant (enhance free radical damage)
Exercise increases need for antioxidants; may help reduce free radical damage, protect cell membranes and reduce post-exercise muscle soreness	Vegetable oils, margarine, oily fish, nuts and seeds, egg yolk, avocado	Toxicity is rare
Low oestrogen in female athletes with amenorrhoea increases bone loss and need for calcium	Milk and dairy products, sardines, dark green leafy vegetables, pulses, nuts and seeds	High intakes may interfere with absorption of other minerals. Take with magnesium and vitamin D.
Female athletes may need more to compensate for menstrual losses	Meat and offal, wholegrain cereals, fortified breakfast cereals, pulses, green leafy vegetables	Constipation, stomach discomfort. Avoid unnecessary supplementation – may increase free radical damage
Exercise increases need for antioxidants; may help immune function	Eggs, wholegrain cereals, meat, milk and dairy products	Interferes with absorption of iron and copper

Magnesium	300 mg (men) 270 mg (women) SUL= 400 mg	Healthy bones; muscle and nerve function; cell formation
Potassium	3500 mg SUL = 3700mg	Fluid balance; muscle and nerve function
Selenium	75 ug (men) 60 ug (women) SUL = 350 ug	Antioxidant which helps protect against heart disease and cancer

Notes:

mg= milligrams (1000 mg = 1 gram)

ug = micrograms (1000 ug = 1 mg)

*The amount needed is given as the Reference Nutrient Intake (RNI, Department of Health, 1991). This is the amount of a nutrient that should cover the needs of 97 per cent of the population. Athletes may need more.

SUL = Safe Upper Limit recommended by the Expert Group on Vitamins and Minerals, an independent advisory committee to the Food Standards Agency.

NITRIC OXIDE SUPPLEMENTS

What are they?

The active ingredient in Nitric Oxide (NO) supplements is L-arginine, a non-essential amino acid, made naturally in the body. It is usually sold as arginine alpha keto-glutarate (A-AKG) and arginine keto iso-caproate (A-KIC). Supplements are marketed to bodybuilders for promoting and prolonging muscle pumps and increasing lean body mass and strength.

May improve recovery after strength training Increased aerobic capacity	Cereals, fruit, vegetables, milk	May cause diarrhoea
May help prevent cramp	Fruit, vegetables, cereals	Excess is excreted
Exercise increases free radical production	Cereals, vegetables, dairy products, meat, eggs	Nausea, vomiting, hair loss

What do they do?

Arginine is an amino acid that is readily converted to NO in the body. NO is a gas that is involved in vasodilation, which is the process that increases blood flow to muscles, allowing better delivery of nutrients and oxygen. The idea behind the NO-boosting supplements is to use L-arginine, A-AKG and A-KIC to increase the production of NO to bring a greater influx of nutrients and oxygen to the muscles, causing a better pump when lifting weights, and increased recovery and muscle growth.

Little research supports these assertions directly, but arginine's NO-boosting effect improves muscle growth in young rats, whereas KIC and AKG have muscle-building or muscle-supporting effects of their own.

Do you need them?

It's certainly plausible that these NO supplements may improve muscle pump when lifting weights. However, more research needs to be done to confirm whether they increase muscle mass and strength in humans.

Are there any side effects?

Side effects are unlikely from the doses recommended on the supplement label. Arginine supplements have been used safely with heart disease patients in doses up to 20 g a day.

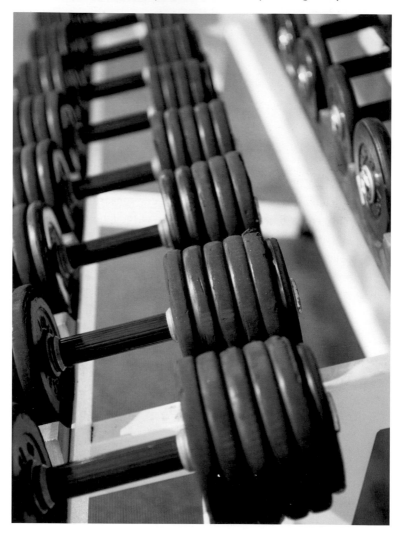

PROTEIN SUPPLEMENTS

What's in them?

Protein supplements can be divided into three main categories: protein powders (which you mix with milk or water into a shake), ready-to-drink shakes and high-protein bars. They may contain whey protein, casein, soy protein or a mixture of these.

What do they do?

They provide a concentrated source of protein to supplement your usual food intake. Whey protein is derived from milk and contains high levels of the essential amino acids, which are readily digested, absorbed and retained by the body for muscle repair (see 'Whey protein', page 110). Whey protein may also help enhance the immune function. Casein, also derived from milk, provides a slower-digested protein, as well as high levels of amino acids (see 'Casein', page 50). It may help protect against muscle breakdown during intense training. Soy protein is less widely used in supplements, but is a good option for vegans and people with high cholesterol levels – 25 g of soya protein daily (as part of a diet low in saturated fat) can help reduce cholesterol levels.

Do you need them?

Most regular exercisers can get enough protein from 2–4 daily portions of meat, chicken, fish, dairy products, eggs and pulses. Vegetarians can meet their protein needs by eating a variety of plant proteins, such as tofu, quorn, beans, lentils, and nuts, each day. However, protein supplements may benefit you if you have particularly high protein requirements (e.g. through strength and power training), you are on a calorie-restricted diet, or you cannot consume enough protein from food alone (e.g. through a vegetarian or vegan diet). Estimate your daily protein intake from food and compare that with your protein requirement. Experts recommend an intake between 1.2 and 1.4 g per kg of body weight per day for endurance athletes, and between 1.4 and 1.8 g per kg body weight per day for strength athletes. For example, a strength athlete weighing 80 kg may need as much as 144 g protein a day. This may be difficult to get from food alone. If there is a consistent shortfall, consider adding a supplement.

HOW TO CHOOSE THE RIGHT PROTEIN BAR

- For rapid refuelling, go for a bar that contains between two to three times as much carbohydrate as protein.
- Check the bar contains whey protein, soy or casein protein, rather than hydrolysed gelatine (which is made from the hooves of cows and horses!).
- Steer clear of bars that list corn syrup, sugar syrup, glucose or sweeteners as their main ingredients.
- Check that the bar contains no more than 5 g of fat per 200 calories and doesn't include palm kernel oil or hydrogenated fat.

Are there any side effects?

An excessive intake of protein, whether from food or supplements, is not harmful but offers no health or performance advantage. Concerns about excess protein harming the liver and kidneys or causing calcium loss from the bones have been disproved.

More about protein supplements

Including protein in your post-workout meal together with carbohydrate can enhance recovery. Researchers at the University of Texas, Austin, USA, have found that a ratio of about one part protein to three parts carbohydrate promotes faster glycogen refuelling, muscle repair and growth compared with carbohydrate alone. For example, consume a protein shake with a couple of bananas or a bowl of cereal.

PRO-HORMONES/PRE-HORMONES/STEROID PRECURSORS/TESTOSTERONE BOOSTERS

What are they?

Pre-hormone supplements include dehydroepiandrosterone (DHEA), androstenedione ('andro') and norandrostenedione, weak androgenic steroid compounds. They are produced naturally in the body and converted into testosterone. Supplements are marketed to bodybuilders and other athletes for increased strength and muscle mass.

What do they do?

Manufacturers claim the supplements will increase testosterone levels in the body and produce similar muscle-building effects to anabolic steroids, but without the side effects. However, these claims are not supported by research. For example, researchers at Iowa State University, USA, found that andro and DHEA supplements combined with a weight-training programme raised levels of androstenedione in the blood, but failed to elevate testosterone or increase strength or muscle mass. Higher doses than those recommended on supplement labels may raise testosterone, but there's no evidence that this results in greater muscle mass or strength.

Do you need them?

It is unlikely that pro-hormones work and they may produce unwanted side effects (*see* page 106). Most athletic associations, including the International Olympic Committee (IOC), ban pro-hormones. What's more, their contents cannot always be guaranteed. In tests carried out by the IOC laboratory in Cologne, Germany, 15 per cent of the supplements contained substances that would lead to a failed drugs test, including nandrolone, despite them not being listed on the label. Pre-hormones are highly controversial supplements and, despite the rigorous marketing, there is no research to prove the testosterone-building claims.

Are there any side effects?
Studies have found that pre-hormones increase oestrogen (which can lead to gynecomastia, male breast development) and decrease HDL (good cholesterol) levels. Reduced HDL carries a greater heart disease risk. Other side effects include acne, enlarged prostate and water retention. Some supplements include anti-oestrogen substances, such as chrysin (dihydroxy-flavone), to counteract the side effects, but there is no evidence that they work either.

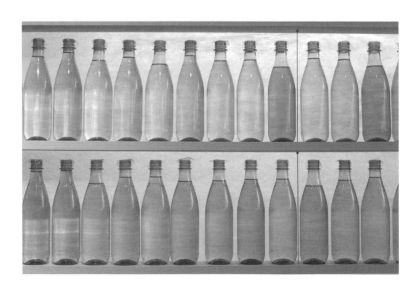

SPORTS DRINKS

(*See* also 'Energy drinks', page 64)

What are they?

Sports drinks fall into two categories: (a) fluid replacement drinks containing up to 8 g carbohydrate per 100 ml, and (b) energy drinks containing 12–20 g carbohydrate per 100 ml. Both categories provide water, carbohydrate (in the form of sucrose, glucose, fructose and maltodextrin) and electrolytes (sodium and potassium), and are designed to replace body fluids more rapidly than plain water. A growing number of recovery drinks are available, which contain small amounts of protein or amino acids (around 1–2 g per 100 ml).

What do they do?

The sugars and maltodextrin (complex carbohydrates derived from cornstarch, consisting of 8–20 glucose units per molecule) in sports drinks help speed the absorption of water from your gut into your bloodstream. The carbohydrate concentration may be either **isotonic** – the same concentration as body fluids – or **hypotonic** – more dilute than body fluids. Research from the University of Texas, USA, found that drinking water during one hour of cycling improved performance by 6 per cent compared with no water, but drinking a sugar-containing drink resulted in a 12 per cent improvement on performance. The purpose of sodium in sports drinks is to stimulate drinking (salt makes you thirsty) and help your body better retain the fluid. Recovery drinks containing low concentrations of protein have been shown to increase fluid retention by 15 per cent compared with regular sports drinks and 40 per cent compared with plain water.

Do you need them?

If you are working out continually for longer than 60 minutes, a sports drink instead of water may help you keep going longer or workout harder. Drink between 500 ml–1 l per hour. If you haven't eaten for more than 4 hours, try a pre-workout sports drink. If you are training between 1 and 2 hours, choose fluid replacement drinks containing less than 8 g sugar per 100 ml. For intense workouts lasting longer than 2 hours, choose an energy drink based on maltodextrin. For a less expensive alternative, try mixing fruit juice with equal quantities of water. This produces an isotonic drink with around 6 g sugar per 100 ml. Add a pinch (one-quarter of a teaspoon) of ordinary salt if you sweat heavily.

Are there any side effects?
Side effects are unlikely, provided you stick to the recommended dilution on the label. Avoid caffeine- and ephedrine-containing drinks if you are sensitive to their side effects.

TAURINE
What is it?
Taurine is a non-essential amino acid produced naturally in the body. It is also found in meat, fish, eggs and milk. It is the second most abundant amino acid in muscle tissue. Taurine is sold as a single supplement, but more commonly as an ingredient in certain protein drinks, creatine-based products and sports drinks. It is marketed to athletes for increasing muscle mass and reducing muscle tissue breakdown during intense exercise.

What does it do?
Taurine has multiple roles in the body, including brain and nervous system function, blood pressure regulation, fat digestion, absorption of fat-soluble vitamins and control of blood cholesterol levels. It is used as a supplement because it is thought to decrease muscle breakdown during exercise. The theory

behind taurine is that it may act in a similar way to insulin, transporting amino acids and sugar from the bloodstream into muscle cells. This would cause an increase in cell volume, triggering protein synthesis and decreasing protein breakdown.

Do you need it?

Intense exercise depletes taurine levels in the body, but there is no sound research to support the claims for taurine supplements. As you can obtain taurine from food (animal protein sources) there appears to be no convincing reason to recommend taking the supplements for athletic performance or muscle gain.

Are there any side effects?

Taurine is harmless in the amounts found in protein and creatine supplements. Very high doses of single supplements may cause toxicity.

TRIBULUS TERRESTIS

What is it?

Tribulus terrestis is a herb, known also as the puncture vine. It is sold as a single supplement, as well as being an ingredient of wider spectrum pro-hormone supplements (see 'Pro-hormones', page 105) marketed for increasing testosterone levels and muscle mass in bodybuilders and power athletes. It is sometimes also marketed as a herbal treatment for impotence.

What does it do?

In theory, tribulus increases testosterone levels indirectly by raising blood levels of another hormone, luteinising hormone (LH). LH is a hormone produced by the pituitary gland and helps to regulate natural testosterone production and serum levels.

However, there has been very little research conducted on the effectiveness of tribulus elevating testosterone levels. Some studies suggest that it can increase testosterone levels 30–50 per cent above baseline levels – but still well within the normal range. No studies have shown it to boost testosterone levels above normal levels or to improve body composition. In one study, 15 resistance-trained males took either a placebo or a large dose of tribulus (1.5 mg per pound of body weight per day) for 2 months. Results showed no changes in body weight, percentage fat, total muscle mass or muscle strength related to tribulus supplementation.

Do you need it?

Due to the lack of scientific support for this supplement, tribulus cannot be recommended for boosting muscle mass. However, as an ingredient in a supplement blend, it may be helpful for males with reduced testosterone levels, such as athletes at risk for overtraining syndrome, and in those individuals on a prolonged low-calorie diet.

Are there any side effects?

Tribulus can increase levels of the female hormone estradiol, which can lead to male breast development – not exactly a desirable effect!

WHEY PROTEIN

What is it?

Whey is a popular ingredient in protein supplements and meal replacement products. It is derived from milk using either a process called micro-filtration (the whey proteins are physically extracted by a microscopic filter) or by ion-exchange (the whey proteins are extracted by taking advantage of their electrical charges).

What does it do?

Whey has a higher concentration of essential amino acids than milk (around 50 per cent), about half (23–25 per cent) of which are branched-chain amino acids, which may help minimise muscle protein breakdown during and immediately after high-intensity exercise. Whey has a higher biological value than most other protein sources. It is digested and absorbed relatively rapidly, making it useful for promoting post-exercise recovery. Research at McGill University, Canada, suggests that the amino acids in whey protein also stimulate glutathione production in the body. Glutathione is a powerful antioxidant and also helps support the immune system. This is particularly useful during periods of intense training when the immune system is suppressed. Whey protein may also help to stimulate muscle growth by increasing insulin-like growth factor-1 (IGF-1) production – a powerful anabolic hormone made in the liver, which enhances protein manufacture in muscles.

Do you need it?

Intense training increases the body's requirement for protein – it is essential for muscle growth, repair and recovery. Experts recommend 1.4–1.8 g per kg body weight per day for strength athletes (equivalent to 112–144 g daily for an 80 kg athlete), which may be difficult for some athletes to obtain solely from food sources. Whey has an especially high concentration of essential amino acids that are important for building and main-taining muscle, and, as a major ingredient in many protein powders and meal replacement products, can be useful for supplementing your food intake if you are engaged in intense strength training.

Are there any side effects?

High intakes are unlikely to have any harmful effect in healthy people.

ZMA (ZINC MONOMETHIONINE ASPARTATE AND MAGNESIUM ASPARTATE)

What is it?

ZMA is a supplement that combines zinc, magnesium, vitamin B6 and aspartate in a specific formula. It is marketed to body-builders and strength athletes as a testosterone booster.

What does it do?

Manufacturers claim that ZMA can boost testosterone production by up to 30 per cent, strength by up to 11 per cent, muscle mass and recovery after exercise. The basis for these claims is that the supplement corrects underlying zinc and/or magnesium deficiencies, thus 'normalising' various body processes and improving testosterone levels. Zinc is needed for growth, cell reproduction and testosterone production. In theory, a deficiency may reduce the body's anabolic hormone levels and adversely affect muscle mass and strength. Magnesium helps reduce levels of the stress hormone cortisol (high levels are produced during periods of intense training), which would otherwise promote muscle breakdown. A magnesium deficiency may increase cata-bolism. ZMA supplements may therefore help increase anabolic hormone levels and keep high levels of cortisol at bay by correcting a zinc and magnesium deficiency.

Do you need it?

Strength and power athletes during periods of intense training may benefit from ZMA, but only if dietary levels of zinc and magnesium are low. Don't expect dramatic strength gains, though. You can obtain zinc from wholegrains, including wholemeal bread, nuts, beans and lentils. Magnesium is found in wholegrains, vegetables, fruit and milk.

Are there any side effects?

Do not exceed the safe upper limit of 25 mg daily for zinc; 400 mg daily for magnesium. High levels of zinc – more than 50 mg – can interfere with the absorption of iron and other minerals, leading to iron-deficiency. Check the zinc content of any other supplement you may be taking.

FURTHER INFORMATION

WEBSITES

Australian Institute of Sport

www.ausport.gov.au

The official website of the Australian Institute of Sport provides factsheets on a wide range of sports-nutrition topics, including advice for different sports.

Drug Information Database (DID)

www.didglobal.com

An online service that provides athletes and their support personnel with fast and accurate information about which drugs and other substances are prohibited under the rules of sport.

Food Standards Agency

www.eatwell.gov.uk

The website of the government's Food Standards Agency has news of nutrition surveys, nutrition and health information.

Gatorade Sports Science Institute

www.gssiweb.com

This website provides in-depth articles and reports on sports nutrition, training, psychology, sports injuries and medical conditions, all written by scientists.

Health Supplements Information Service

www.hsis.org

Provides good information on vitamins, minerals and supplements.

Nutritional Supplements Knowledgebase

www.nutros.com

This website contains a large up-to-date database on nutritional supplements.

Runner's World

www.runnersworld.co.uk

The website of the UK edition of *Runner's World* magazine provides an extensive library of excellent articles on nutrition, training and sports injuries, and sports nutrition product reviews.

SupplementWatch

www.supplementwatch.com

A useful website providing impartial advice and information about supplements, including sports supplements and health concerns, product reviews, news and product recommendations.

thefitmap

www.thefitmap.co.uk

A website providing sound information about nutrition and fitness (among other topics), including articles on sports nutrition, sports supplements and a useful directory of websites and retail outlets selling sports supplements.

BOOKS

Antonio J. and Stout J. *Supplements for endurance athletes* (Human Kinetics, 2002)

Antonio J. and Stout J. *Supplements for strength-power athletes* (Human Kinetics, 2002)

Bean, A. *The Complete Guide to Sports Nutrition*, 5th edition (A&C Black, 2006)

Bean, A. *Food For Fitness*, 3rd edition (A & C Black, 2007)

USEFUL ADDRESSES

British Dietetic Association
5th floor, Charles House
148–9 great Charles Street
Queensway
Birmingham, B3 3HT
www.bda.uk.com

British Nutrition Foundation
High Holborn House
London, WC1V 6RQ
www.nutrition.org.uk/

Dietitians in Sport and Exercise Nutrition (DISEN)
PO Box 22360
London, W13 9FL
www.disen.org/

Food Standards Agency
Room 621, Hannibal house
PO Box 30080
London, SE1 6YA
www.foodstandards.gov.uk

The Nutrition Society
10 Cambridge court
210 Shepherds Bush Road
London, W6 7NJ
www.nutritionsociety.org/

Vegetarian Society
Parkdale
Dunham Road
Altrincham
Cheshire, WA14 4QG
www.vegsoc.org

INDEX

ABOUT THE AUTHOR

Anita Bean has an inspiring approach to nutrition and fitness. Her practical style has made her one of the UK's most respected sports nutritionists. She is an accomplished sportsperson and author of 19 best-selling books including *The Complete Guide to Sports Nutrition* and *The Complete Guide to Strength Training*. Winner of two major achievement awards in sports nutrition she features regularly in the media, including *Runners World*, *Zest and Men's Health*. She also broadcasts on TV and radio.

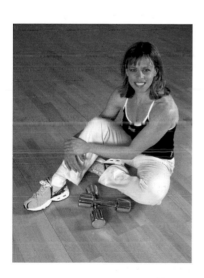

OTHER BOOKS FROM
ANITA BEAN

The Complete Guide to Sports Nutrition, 5th edition (A&C Black, 2006)

The Complete Guide to Sports Nutrition is the definitive practical handbook for anyone wanting a performance advantage. This fully updated and revised edition incorporates the latest cutting edge research. Written by one of the country's most respected sports nutritionists, it provides the latest information to help you succeed.

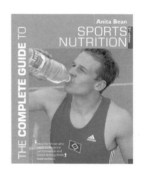

Food for Fitness, 3rd edition (A&C Black, 20067)

Food for Fitness is the bible for anyone who is serious about their sport, health and fitness. This new edition has seen a complete overhaul of the book – radically improving the design and adding lots of new material.

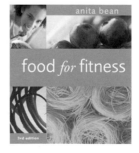

The book is now in full colour and contains lots of engaging fact boxes and top tips from leading sportspeople and athletes, as well as high quality photography.